Recent Trends in
Microbial
Biotechnology

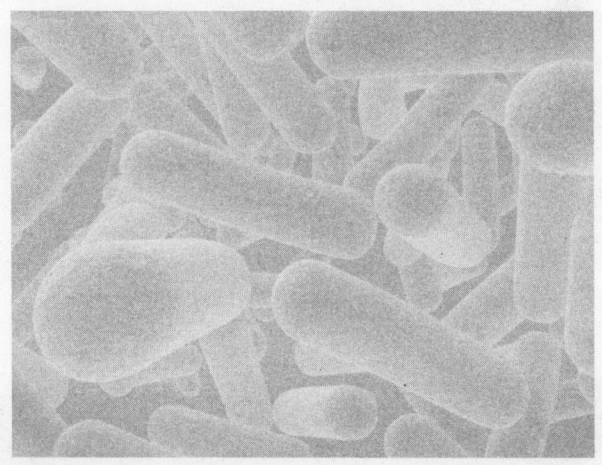

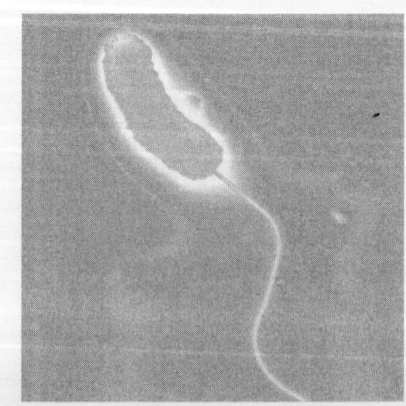

Recent Trends in
Microbial
Biotechnology

Padma Singh PhD, FBS, FAPSI

Associate Professor
Department of Microbiology
Girls' Campus
Gurukul Kangri University
Haridwar
Uttarakhand, India

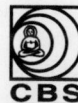

CBS Publishers & Distributors Pvt Ltd

New Delhi • Bengaluru • Chennai • Kochi • Pune
• Hyderabad • Kolkata • Mumbai • Nagpur • Patna

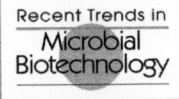

ISBN: 978-81-239-2212-6

Copyright © Author and Publisher

First Edition: 2013

Published by Satish Kumar Jain and produced by Vinod K. Jain for

CBS Publishers & Distributors Pvt Ltd

4819/XI Prahlad Street, 24 Ansari Road, Daryaganj, New Delhi 110 002, India.

Ph: 23289259, 23266861, 23266867   Fax: 011-23243014   Website: www.cbspd.com
e-mail: delhi@cbspd.com; cbspubs@airtelmail.in

Corporate Office: 204 FIE, Industrial Area, Patparganj, Delhi 110 092

Ph: 4934 4934   Fax: 4934 4935   e-mail: publishing@cbspd.com; publicity@cbspd.com

Branches

- **Bengaluru:** Seema House 2975, 17th Cross, K.R. Road,
  Banasankari 2nd Stage, Bengaluru 560 070, Karnataka
  Ph: +91-80-26771678/79   Fax: +91-80-26771680   e-mail: bangalore@cbspd.com
- **Chennai:** 20, West Park Road, Shenoy Nagar, Chennai 600 030, Tamil Nadu
  Ph: +91-44-26260666, 26208620   Fax: +91-44-42032115   e-mail: chennai@cbspd.com
- **Kochi:** 36/14 Kalluvilakam, Lissie Hospital Road, Kochi 682 018, Kerala
  Ph: +91-484-4059061-65   Fax: +91-484-4059065   e-mail: kochi@cbspd.com
- **Pune:** Bhuruk Prestige, Sr. No. 52/12/2+1+3/2 Narhe, Haveli
  (Near Katraj-Dehu Road Bypass), Pune 411 041, Maharashtra
  Ph: +91-20-64704058, 64704059, 32342277   Fax: +91-20-24300160   e-mail: pune@cbspd.com

Representatives

- **Hyderabad** 0-9885175004   • **Kolkata** 0-9831437309, 0-9051152362   • **Mumbai** 0-9833017933
- **Nagpur** 0-9021734563   • **Patna** 0-9334159340

Printed at India Binding House, Noida, UP

List of Contributors

Arya Garima
Department of Microbiology
Kanya Gurukul Girls' Campus
Gurukul Kangri Vishwavidyalaya (GKV)
Haridwar 249407

Bhanot Leena
Department of Biotechnology
Lovely Professional University
Phagwara
Punjab 144003

Bahuguna Ashutosh
Department of Biotechnology
Modern Institute of Technology
Dhalwala
Rishikesh 249201

Chauhan Mamta
Department of Microbiology
Kanya Gurukul Girls' Campus
GKV
Haridwar 2494071

Dangwal Koushalya
Department of Biotechnology
Modern Institute of Technology
Dhalwala
Rishikesh 249201

Dhewa Tejpal
Department of Microbiology
Dolphin (PG) Institute of Biomedical and
Natural Sciences
Manduwala
Dehradun 248007

Joshi Shailesh K
Department of Microbiology
Dolphin (PG) Institute of Biomedical and
Natural Sciences
Manduwala
Dehradun 248007

Kaushik Surbhi
Department of Microbiology
Kanya Gurukul Girls' Campus
GKV, Haridwar 249407

Lily Madhuri K
Department of Biotechnology
Modern Institute of Technology
Dhalwala
Rishikesh 249201

Malik Tripti
Department of Microbiology
Dolphin (PG) Institute of Biomedical
and Natural Sciences
Manduwala
Dehradun 248007

Pant Shailja
Department of Microbiology
Dolphin (PG) Institute of Biomedical and
Natural Sciences
Manduwala, Dehradun 248007

Parihar Leena
Department of Biotechnology
Lovely Professional University
Phagwara, Punjab 144003

Parihar Pradeep
Department of Biotechnology
Lovely Professional University
Phagwara, Punjab 144003

Singh Padma
Department of Microbiology
Kanya Gurukul Girls' Campus
GKV, Haridwar 249407

Sisodia Yamini Singh
Department of Biotechnology
Lovely Professional University
Phagwara, Punjab 144003

Soni Deepti
Department of Biotechnology
Lovely Professional University
Phagwara
Punjab 144003

Sood Gunjan
Department of Biotechnology
Lovely Professional University
Phagwara
Punjab 144003

Srivastava Deepika

Department of Microbiology
Kanya Gurukul Girls' Campus
GKV, Haridwar 249407

Trivedi Bhavya

Department of Microbiology
Kanya Gurukul Girls' Campus
GKV
Haridwar 249407

Preface

Microbiology is emerging as the key biological science in which unseen microorganisms are at the centre stage of revolution called *biotechnology*. The subject has tremendous scope of development in future. Microbial biotechnology is the application of scientific and engineering principles to the processing of materials by biological agents to provide goods, etc. Microbial biotechnology may have a profound effect on the world economy over the next two decades. Innovations emerging in the food and pharmaceutical sectors point to the enormous potential of biotechnology to provide diverse new products including disease-resistant plants, natural pesticides, environmental remediation technologies and novel therapeutic agents, etc.

The present book provides an authoritative review account of many aspects of current interest and progress in the field of microbial biotechnology that have been made in recent past. It includes 12 chapters prepared by subject experts on different aspects of microbial technology. Topics covering role of vesicular-arbiscular mycorrhizae (VAM) and symbiotic N_2-fixation in microbial technology, lactic acid bacteria (LAB), actinomycetes as antibiotics, medicinal importance of spices, gene diversity and genomic evolution, bacterial communications, biotechnological interventions of new antimicrobials, biofuel production, biodeterioration of buildings, nanotechnology and bioinformaticas, etc. have been especially included to project their use in the 21st century. Each chapter has been written in explanatory style combined with an extensive cross-referencing system. The book covers the topics of postgraduate curriculum as well as for those in research field. I have tried to maintain a balance between the fundamental and applied microbiology so that strong continuum of research development from basics to the applied can be established.

I am confident that the book will be widely accepted by all the students, teachers and researchers in the field of microbiology and biotechnology.

Padma Singh

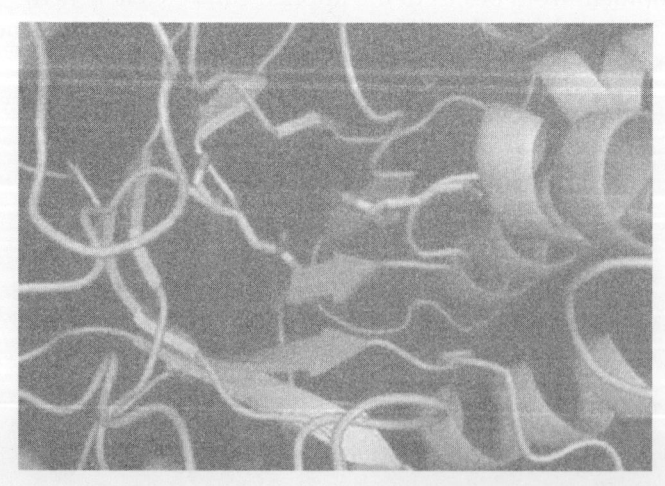

Acknowledgements

I am thankful to all the contributors who have contributed their valuable chapters and for their cooperation in compiling useful information on various facets of microbial biotechnology. I have been constantly encouraged by my colleagues for this so I am indebted to them in general. Thanks are due to my research scholars and technical assistant for helping me in preparation of this book. I record my sincere gratitude to my family for their full cooperation and moral support during the preparation of this book.

I highly appreciate the all round cooperation and support of Mr YN Arjuna, Senior Director, CBS Publishers & Distributors Pvt Ltd, for publishing this book with patience, care and interest.

Padma Singh

Acknowledgements

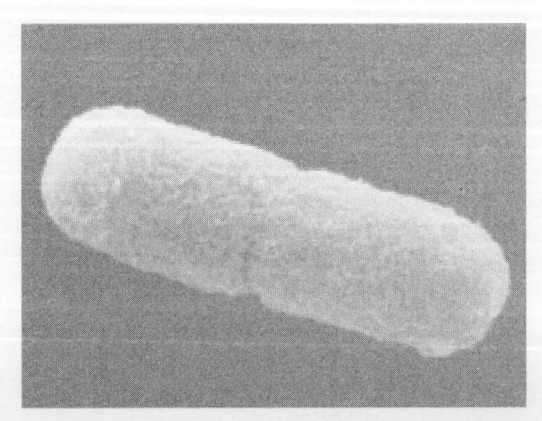

Contents

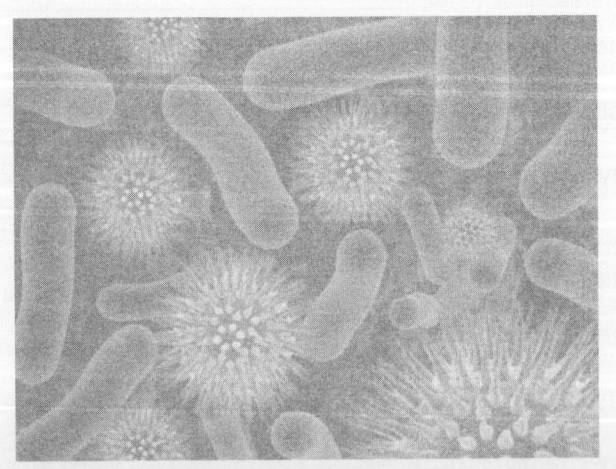

1

Role of Vesicular-arbuscular Mycorrhiza (VAM) in Microbial Biotechnology

Leena Bhanot • Leena Parihar

INTRODUCTION

Mycorrhiza is a symbiotic association between a fungus and the roots of a plant. In a mycorrhizal association, the fungus colonizes the roots of a host plant, either intracellularly or extracellularly. They are an important part of soil life. The benefits afforded plants from mycorrhizal symbioses can be characterized either agronomically by increased growth and yield or ecologically by improved fitness (i.e. reproductive ability). In either case, the benefit accrues primarily because mycorrhizal fungi form a critical linkage between plant roots and the soil. Mycorrhizal fungi usually proliferate both in the root and in the soil. The soil-borne or extra-matrical hyphae take up nutrients from the soil solution and transport them to the root. By this mechanism, mycorrhizae increase the effective absorptive surface area of the plant. In nutrient-poor or moisture-deficient soils, nutrients taken up by the extra-matrical hyphae can lead to improved plant growth and reproduction. As a result, mycorrhizal plants are often more competitive and better able to tolerate environmental stresses than are non-mycorrhizal plants (Harrison MJ 2005).

This mutualistic association provides the fungus with relatively constant and direct access to mono- or dimeric carbohydrates, such as glucose and sucrose produced by the plant in photosynthesis. The carbohydrates are translocated from their source location (usually leaves) to the root tissues and then to the fungal partners. In return, the plant gains the use of the Mycelium's very large surface area to absorb water and mineral nutrients from the soil, thus improving the mineral absorption capabilities of the plant roots. Plant roots alone may be incapable of taking up phosphate ions that are immobilized, e.g. in soils with a basic pH. The mycelium of the mycorrhizal fungus can, however, access these phosphorus sources, and make them available to the plants they colonize. The mechanisms of increased absorption are both physical and chemical.

1

Mycorrhizal mycelia are much smaller in diameter than the smallest root, and can explore a greater volume of soil, providing a larger surface area for absorption. Also, the cell membrane chemistry of fungi is different from that of plants. Mycorrhizae are especially beneficial for the plant partner in nutrient-poor soils. Mycorrhizae form a mutualistic relationship with the roots of most plant species and while only a small proportion of all species has been examined, 95% of these plant families are predominantly mycorrhizal. Mycorrhizal relationships have been found in 460 million-year-old Ordovician fossils (Redecker et al. 2000). Since then the fungi have become very specialized so that most cannot survive unless they are in contact with their host plant. Many plants have also become equally dependent on mycorrhizal fungi and without them the plants become stunted and yellow, often due to a lack of phosphorus (Peterson, 2005). The role of mycorrhiza is basically the relationship between the roots of the plant and the soil. So the basic mechanism between soil–plant relationship is as follows.

SOIL–PLANT RELATIONSHIP

Soil–plant relationship includes the following steps.

Movement of Nutrients from the Soil to the Plant Root

For nutrients to be absorbed by plants, they must come in contact with the roots. There are three ways by which this can occur:

1. Mass Flow

Nutrient ions are transported to the root surface via the flow of water. Plants transpire water which causes a gradient that allows water to flow towards the root. If nutrients are in the water, they will be absorbed by the root. Nutrients supplied to plant roots by mass flow: Ca^{+2}, Mg^{+2}, NO_3^-, Cl^-, H_3BO_3.

These nutrients are not held tightly by the soil that is why these nutrients can be supplied by mass flow. Mass flow is most important for nutrients or ions in relative abundance in the soil solution. There are few factors which influence mass flow like soil moisture (drier the soil, less mass flow), size of root system, soil temperature (cooler temperature means less transpiration), etc.

2. Diffusion

Diffusion is the spontaneous migration of substances from regions where their concentration is high to regions where their concentration is low. Ion diffusion occurs in the soil solution. Ions dissolved in the soil solution will move from areas of high concentration to areas of low concentration.

Area around the root of an actively growing plant is depleted of nutrients (low concentration), so nutrients in the soil will migrate towards the root. Nutrients supplied to plant root by diffusion: P and K. These nutrients have a low solubility.

Factors Influencing Diffusion

Concentration gradient–Diffusion rate = Dc × Area × gradient

Dc   = Diffusion coefficient (tortuosity)
Area   = root area
Gradient = concentration gradient

a. *Tortuosity:* The path the diffusion ion must take. Large soil pore and adequate soil moisture decreases tortuosity, so diffusion is easier and occurs more. Small pores (clay soil) and low soil moisture increases tortuosity which makes diffusion more difficult.

b. *Temperature:* Motion of atoms or ions increases with temperature; hence diffusion rates are greater at higher temperatures; cool soil temperatures often limit diffusion rates in Alaska soils.

c. *Chemical and physical properties of the soil:* Lower the pH, the more quickly ions will diffuse.

3. Root Interception

As roots extend through the soil, they continually come in contact with previously unexplored soil. Therefore, root surfaces come in direct contact with nutrients during this displacement process.

Factors Influencing Root Interception

The quantity of nutrients absorbed by root interception is a function of the root volume. Typically, no more than 1% of the soil by volume is ever directly contacted by roots. Ca and Mg are most often intercepted by root contact.

Mycorrhizae can increase nutrient uptake by root interception. Mycorrhizae are a symbiotic association between fungi and the roots of seed plants. This association increases the surface area that roots can extract nutrients from.

Root System Sorption Zone for Mobile and Immobile Nutrients

Mobile nutrients form soluble compounds and do not interact with the soil (i.e. they do not attach to soil particles) and are found in comparatively high concentration in the soil solution. The nutrient sorption zone will be comparatively large. Immobile nutrients are insoluble and attach to the soil particles. The nutrient sorption zone is more localized around the plant roots.

WORKING OF MYCORRHIZAL FUNGI

Mycorrhizal root systems increase the absorptive capacity. The absorbing area of roots increases 10 to 1000 times thereby greatly improving the ability of the plants to utilize the soil resource. Mycorrhizal fungi are able to absorb and transfer all of the major macro-and micro-nutrients necessary for plant growth. Mycorrhizal fungi release powerful chemicals into the soil that dissolve hard to capture nutrients such as phosphorus, iron and other "tightly bound" soil nutrients. This extraction process is particularly important in plant nutrition and explains why non-mycorrhizal plants require high levels of fertility to maintain their health. Mycorrhizal fungi form an intricate web that captures and assimilates nutrients conserving the nutrient capital in soils. In non-mycorrhizal conditions, much of this fertility is wasted or lost from the system.

Mycorrhizal fungi are involved with a wide variety of other activities that benefit plant establishment and growth. The same extensive network of fungal filaments important to nutrient uptake is also important in water uptake and storage. In non-irrigated conditions, mycorrhizal plants are under far less drought stress compared to non-mycorrhizal plants. In a recent study, true fir seedlings treated with mycorrhizal inoculum had 43% less plant moisture stress than non-treated control seedlings on a droughty, difficult to revegetate site. Tree vigour, colour and needle retention were improved with the mycorrhizal treated plants. *Rhizopogon mycorrhizae* were abundant on the roots systems of the treated plants. Numerous studies have shown *Rhizopogon* sp. is an aggressive colonizer in non-irrigated and harsh field conditions. Disease and pathogen suppression is another benefit for a mycorrhizal plant. Mycorrhizal roots have a mantle (a tight, interwoven sock-like covering of dense filaments) that acts as a physical barrier against the invasio of root diseases. In addition, mycorrhizal fungi attack pathogen or disease organisms entering the root zone. For example, excretions of specific antibiotics produced by mycorrhizal fungi immobilize and kill disease organisms. Some mycorrhizal fungi protect pine trees from phytopthora, fusarium and rhizoctonia diseases. In a recent University study, pine trees were purposefully inoculated with the common disease organism—*Fusarium*. Over 90% of the pine trees died. Only the pine trees inoculated with the mycorrhizal fungus *Rhizopogon* survived. Survival rates for *Rhizopogon* treated pines exceeded 95%.

Mycorrhizal fungi also improve soil structure. Mycorrhizal filaments produce humic compounds and organic "glues" (extracellular polysaccharides) that bind soils into aggregates and improve soil porosity.

Soil porosity and soil structure positively influence the growth of plants by promoting aeration, water movement into soil, root growth, and distribution. In sandy or compacted soils, the ability of mycorrhizal fungi to promote soil structure may be more important than the seeking out of nutrients.

IMPORTANCE OF MYCORRHIZAL FUNGI

Natural areas generally contain an array of mycorrhizal fungal species. The proportions and abundance of mycorrhizal species often shift following any disturbance. Not all mycorrhizal fungi have the same capacities and tolerances. Some are better at imparting drought resistance while others may be more effective in protecting against pathogens or have more tolerance to soil temperature extremes. Because of the wide variety of soil, climatic, and biotic conditions characterizing man-made environments, it is improbable that a single mycorrhizal fungus could benefit all host species and adapt to all conditions. For example, the types and activities of mycorrhizal fungi associated with young plants may be quite different from those associated with mature plants. Likewise; mycorrhizal fungi needed to help seedlings establish themselves on difficult sites may differ from those which sustain productivity over a long-lived plant.

Diversity likely provides a buffering capacity not found on sites with only one or few species. The diversity of mycorrhizal fungi formed by a given plant may increase its ability to occupy diverse below-ground niches and survive a range of chemical and physical conditions.

Commercial production of mycorrhizal fungi for practical use has been available in the last decade; however, the importance of mycorrhizal fungi has been evident for some 400 million years. The earliest fossil records of the roots of land plants contain evidence of the fossil remains of mycorrhizal fungi. Scientists now believe that the "marriage" of mycorrhizal fungus and plant played an essential role in the evolutionary step which brought aquatic plants from sea to land. At some point in the evolutionary process, a filament penetrated into the outer cells of a primitive plant root. Once there, it accommodated itself so nicely that a new, more complex entity emerged, the mycorrhiza. The increased absorbing area provided by an elaborate system of fungal filaments allowed aquatic plants to leave the marine environment and exploit a relatively harsh soil environment. In today's man-made environments, plants can be greatly stressed and the relationship between fungus and root is critical. Unnatural conditions such as concrete, asphalt, roadsides, sidewalk cut outs, trenching, drain fields, air pollution, shopping malls, business districts, and suburban developments adversely affect the presence and abundance of mycorrhizal fungi. Man-made environments often suffer from compaction, top soil loss, and the absence of quality organic matter, conditions which reduce the habitat necessary for the mycorrhizal fungus to survive and thrive. Artificial landscapes affect the mycorrhizal relationship in two fundamental ways. First, they isolate the plant from beneficial mycorrhizal fungi available in natural settings and, secondly, they increase plant stress and the need for water, nutrients, and soil structure mediated by their below-ground "partners".

Fortunately, recent advancements in mycorrhizal research and application have made landscape applications with mycorrhiza easy and inexpensive. New products and knowledge result in increased transplant survival and lower long-term maintenance. However, to be successful, the landscape contractor requires an appreciation of fungi beyond itchy toes and moldy bread (Amaranthus, 1993).

TYPES OF MYCORRHIZA

Mycorrhizae are commonly divided into ectomycorrhizae and endomycorrhizae. The two groups are differentiated by the fact that the hyphae of ectomycorrhizal fungi do not penetrate individual cells within the root, while the hyphae of endomycorrhizal fungi penetrate the cell wall and invaginate the cell membrane.

Endomycorrhizae (Fig. 1.1)

Endomycorrhizae are variable and have been further classified as arbuscular, ericoid, arbutoid, monotropoid, and orchid mycorrhizae.

Arbuscular mycorrhizae, or AM (formerly known as vesicular-arbuscular mycorrhizae, or VAM), are mycorrhizae whose hyphae enter into the plant cells, producing structures that are either balloon-like (vesicles) or dichotomously-branching invaginations (arbuscules). The fungal hyphae do not in fact penetrate the protoplast (i.e. the interior of the cell), but invaginate the cell membrane. The structure of the arbuscules greatly increases the contact surface area between the hypha and the cell cytoplasm to facilitate the transfer of nutrients between them. Other structures produced by some AM fungi include vesicles, auxiliary cells, and asexual spores. Vesicles are thin-walled, lipid-filled structures that usually form in intercellular spaces. Their primary function is thought to be for storage; however, vesicles can also serve as reproductive propagules for the fungus. Auxiliary cells are formed in the soil and can be coiled or knobby. The function of these structures is unknown. Reproductive spores can be formed either in the root or more commonly in the soil. Spores produced by fungi forming AM associations are asexual, forming by the differentiation of vegetative hyphae.

Arbuscular mycorrhizae are formed only by fungi in the division Glomeromycota. The taxonomy is further divided into suborders based on the presence of: (i) vesicles in the root and formation of chlamydospores (thick wall, asexual spore) borne from subtending hyphae for the suborder Glomineae or (ii) absence of vesicles in the root and formation of auxiliary cells and azygospores (spores resembling a zygospore but developing asexually from a subtending hypha resulting in a distinct bulbous attachment) in the soil for the suborder Gigasporineae (Fox, 1990). Fossil evidence and DNA sequence analysis suggest that this mutualism appeared 400–460 million years ago, when the first plants were colonizing land. Arbuscular mycorrhizae are found in 85% of all plant families, and occur in many crop species. The hyphae of arbuscular mycorrhizal fungi produce the glycoprotein glomalin, which may be one of the major stores of carbon in the soil. Arbuscular mycorrhizal fungi have (possibly) been asexual for many millions of years and, unusually, individuals can contain many genetically different nuclei (a phenomenon called heterokaryosis).

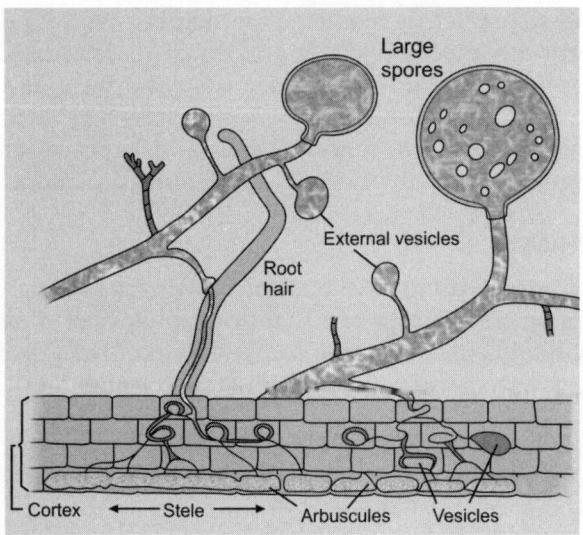

Fig. 1.1: Typical endomycorrhiza including arbuscules, vesicles, and external hyphae with spores (Drawing by FE sanders)

Some of the definitions used are:
- Arbuscules (Fig. 1.2, colour plate 1) – highly branched structures that are the site of nutrient transfer, (Fig. 1.6, colour plate 1) they do not penetrate cell membrane; short-lived structures.
- Vesicles (Fig. 1.3, colour plate 1) – oval-shaped, darkly staining structures that are thought to function as nutrient reservoir.

Alteration of Root Morphology
- VAM do not significantly alter root morphology; fine roots possess root hairs (Fig. 1.4, colour plate 1). EcM alter root morphology; no root hairs; produce a mantle (Fig. 1.5, colour plate 1).

Ectomycorrhizae (EcM)
EcM do not penetrate cell walls of cortex cells. EcM form a puzzled-shape covering of

hyphae over the cortex cells called a Hartig net; site of nutrient transfer, relatively long-lived structures.

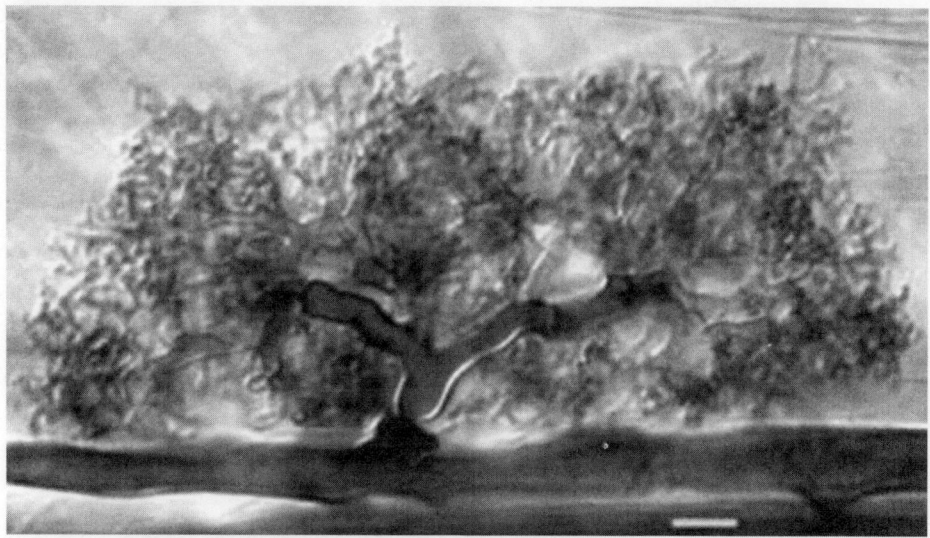

Fig. 1.2: Arbuscules

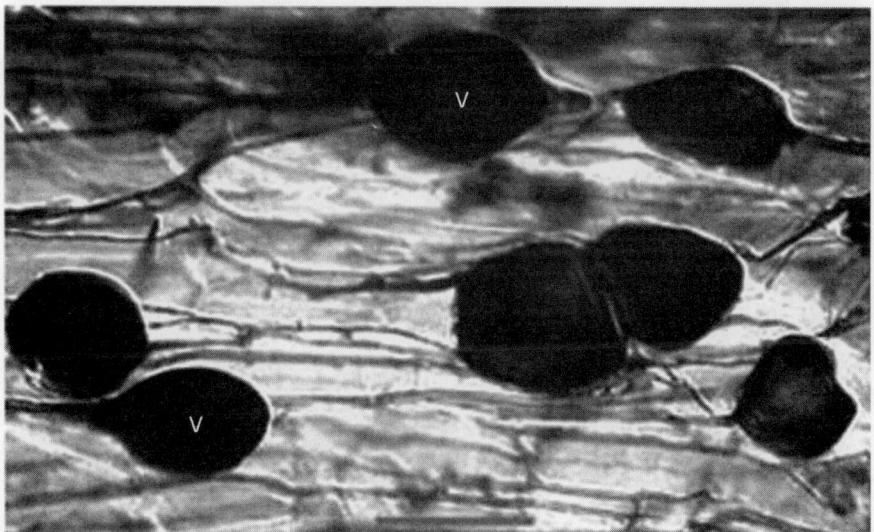

Fig. 1.3: Vesicles

Ectomycorrhizae or EcM, are typically formed between the roots of around 10% of plant families, mostly woody plants including the birch, dipterocarp, eucalyptus, oak, pine, and rose families and fungi belonging to the Basidiomycota, Ascomycota, and Zygomycota. Ectomycorrhizae consist of a hyphal sheath, or mantle, covering the root tip and a hartig net of hyphae surrounding the plant cells within the root cortex.

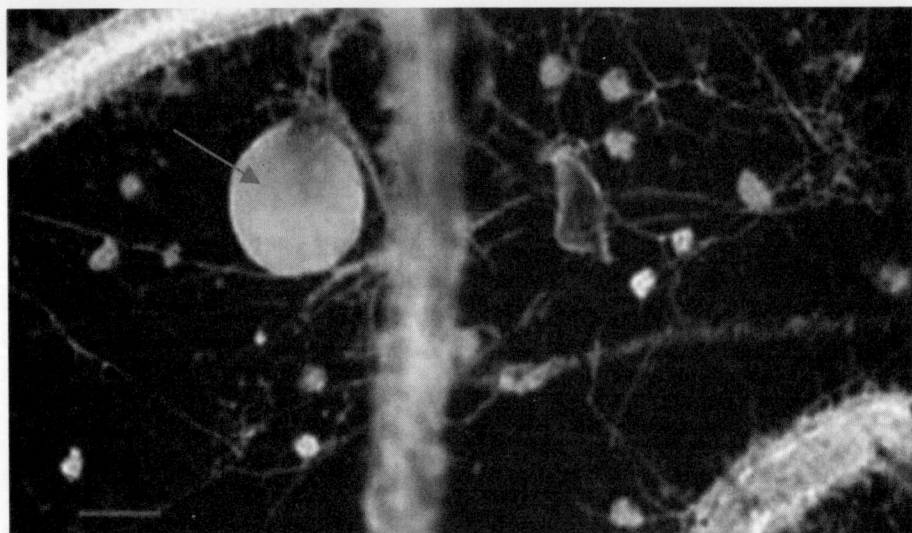

Fig. 1.4: VAM showing fine roots with root hairs

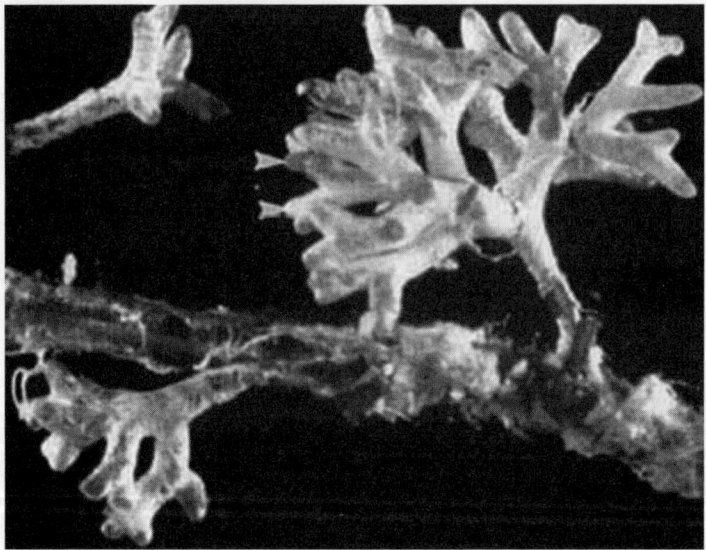

Fig. 1.5: Showing dichotomously branched roots of *Pinus* sp. with ectotrophic fungal mantle around roots

In some cases, the hyphae may also penetrate the plant cells, in that case, the mycorrhiza is called an ectendomycorrhiza. Outside the root, the fungal mycelium forms an extensive network within the soil and leaf litter. Nutrients can be shown to move between different plants through the fungal network (sometimes called the wood wide web). Carbon has been shown to move from birch trees into fir trees thereby promoting succession in ecosystems.

The ectomycorrhizal fungus *Laccaria bicolor* has been found to lure and kill springtails to obtain nitrogen, some of which may then be transferred to the mycorrhizal host

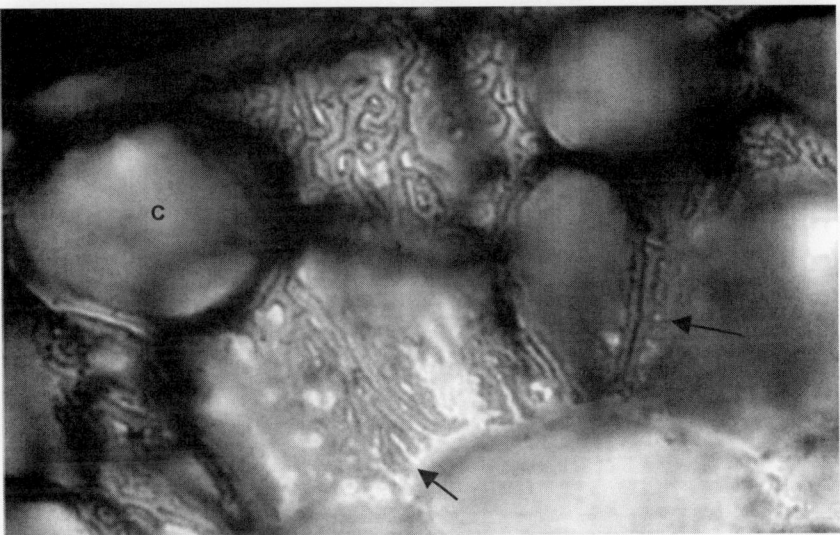

Fig. 1.6: Showing site of nutrient transfer

plant. In a study by Klironomos and Hart, Eastern White Pine inoculated with *L. bicolor* was able to derive up to 25% of its nitrogen from springtails.

An arbuscular mycorrhiza (plural mycorrhizae or mycorrhizas) is a type of mycorrhiza in which the fungus penetrates the cortical cells of the roots of a vascular plant.

Arbuscular mycorrhizae (AMs) are characterized by the formation of unique structures such as arbuscules and vesicles by fungi of the phylum Glomeromycota (AM fungi). AM fungi help plants to capture nutrients such as phosphorus and micronutrients from the soil. It is believed that the development of the arbuscular mycorrhizal symbiosis played a crucial role in the initial colonisation of land by plants and in the evolution of the vascular plants.

It has been said that it is quicker to list the plants that do not form mycorrhizae than those that do. This symbiosis is a highly evolved mutualistic relationship found between fungi and plants, the most prevalent plant symbiosis known, and AM is found in 80% of vascular plant families of today. The tremendous advances in research on mycorrhizal physiology and ecology over the past 40 years have led to a greater understanding of the multiple roles of AMF in the ecosystem. This knowledge is applicable to human endeavors of ecosystem management, ecosystem restoration (Figs 1.7 and 1.8).

GLOMERALES

General characteristic:

1. Coenocytic hyphae
2. Meiosis unknown
3. Lack fruiting structure of basidiomycota and ascomycota
4. No flagellated state in life cycle, obligate symbionts
5. Endomycorrhizae or vesicular-arbuscular mycorrhiza (VAM), symbiosis with cyanobacteria (geosiphon with nostoc) [Fig. 1.15, colour plate 3]

6. Often referred to as "VAM fungi" because they form vesicles and arbuscules

7. Classification includes three families of six genera which are as follows.

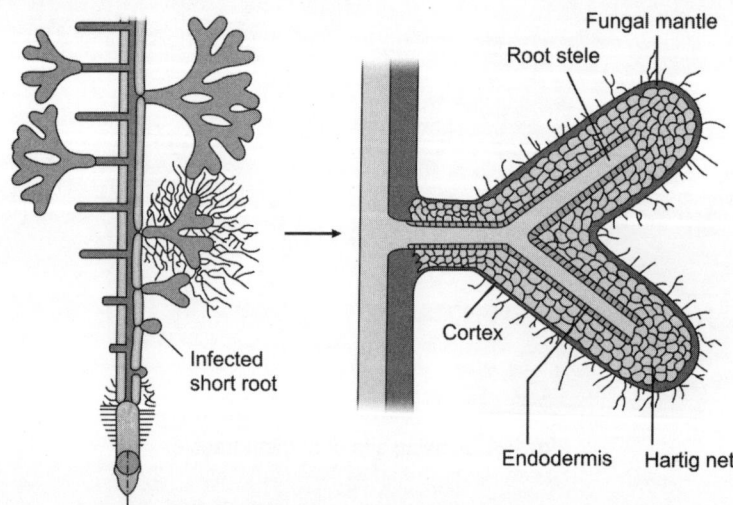

Fig. 1.7: Ectomycorrhizal root: Note the developmental progression of mycorrhizal roots on the left-hand picture. The roots infected with ectomycorrhizae fungi are swollen and branch dichotomously.

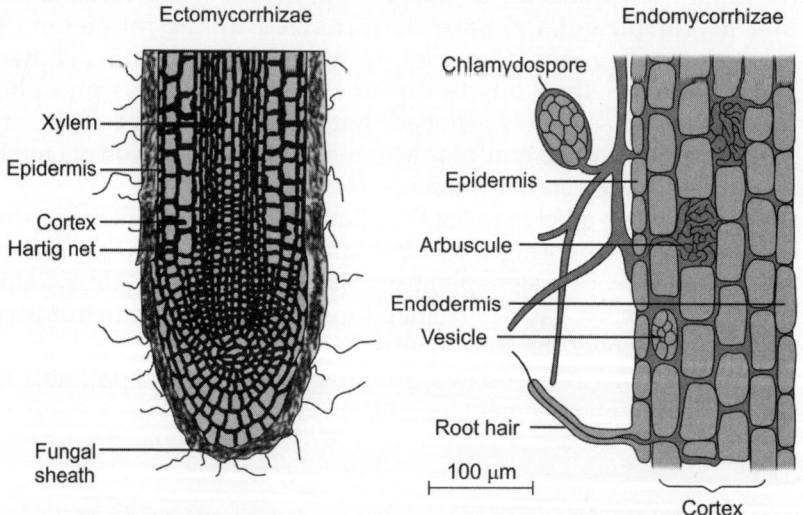

Fig.1.8: Comparison of ectomycorrhizae (left) with endomycorrhizae (right)

Gigasporaceae

Gigaspora and scutellospora (Fig. 1.9, colour plate 1): Only arbuscules in the roots of their mycorrhizal partners auxiliary cells are produced in the soil along with structures called "azygospores"

Azygospore: Term used for spores that are produced on a hypha that resembles the gametangial hypha of some zygomycota. But, meiosis has never been documented in glomerales.

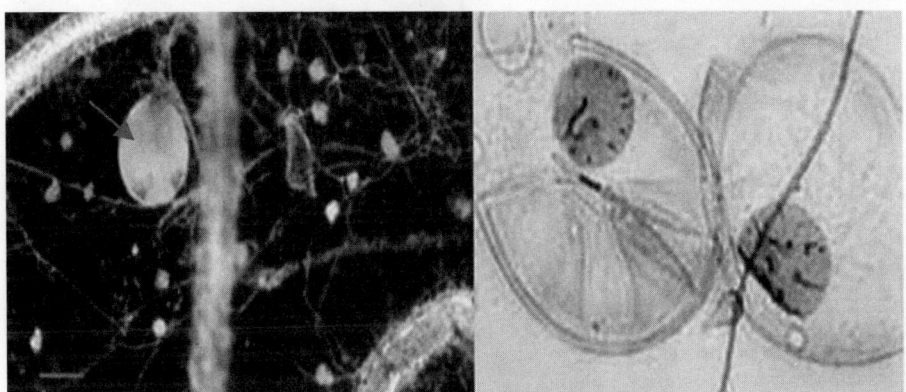

Fig. 1.9: *Gigaspora* and *scutellospora*

Acaulosporaceae: It produces "chlamydospores" in the soil either singly or in sporocarps and spores of both these genera arise from a hypha that subtends. It is a swollen, sac-like structure; "sporiferous saccule" (Figs 1.10 and 1.11, colour plate 2) Acaulospora the spore forms laterally on the subtending hypha and *Entrophospora* spore develops within the neck of the hypha.

• *Entrophospora* spore develops within the neck of the hypha (Fig. 1.12, colour plate 2).

• Glomaceae (Figs 1.13 and 1.14, colour plates 2 and 3)

Recently discovered: Glomeralean fungus symbiotic with a *Cyanobacterium* (Fig. 1.15, colour plate 3).

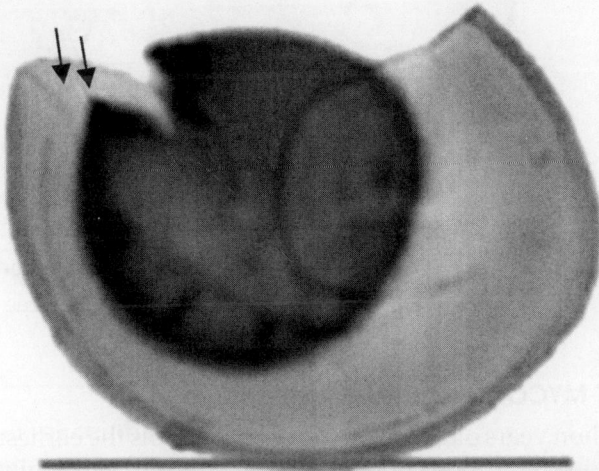

Fig. 1.10: Sporiferous saccule

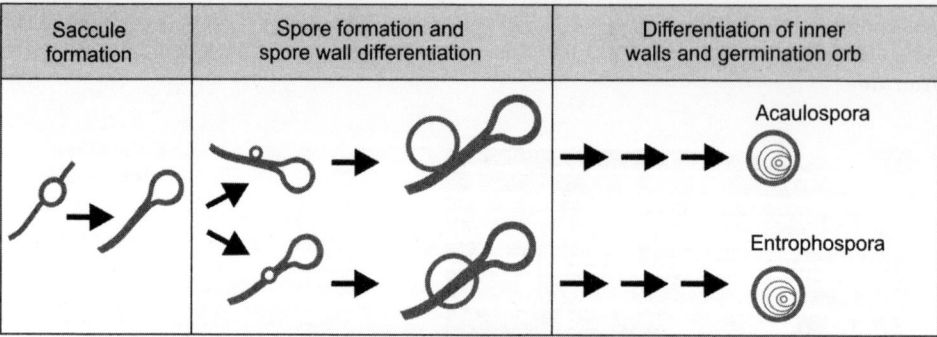

Fig. 1.11: Showing saccule formation

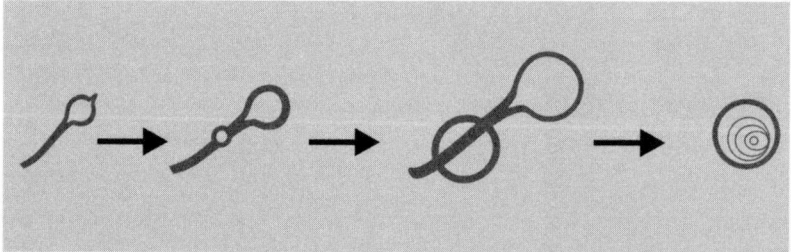

Fig. 1.12: Showing spore development in *Entrophospora*

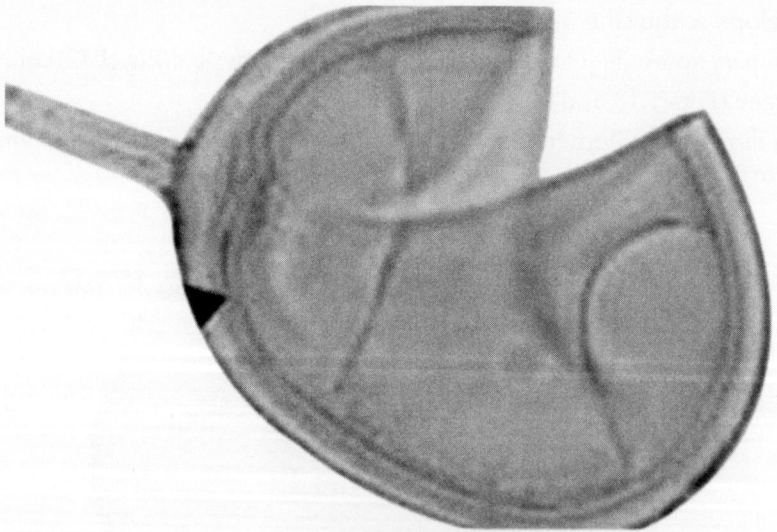

Fig. 1.13: *Glomus*

OCCURRENCE OF MYCORRHIZAL ASSOCIATIONS

At around 400 million years old, the Rhynie chert contains the earliest fossil assemblage yielding plants preserved in sufficient detail to detect mycorrhizae—and they are indeed observed in the stems of Aglaophyton major.

Plate 1

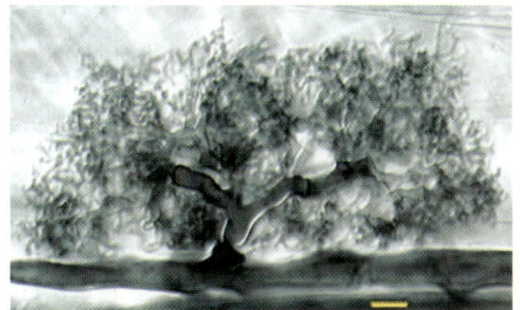

Fig. 1.2: Arbuscules

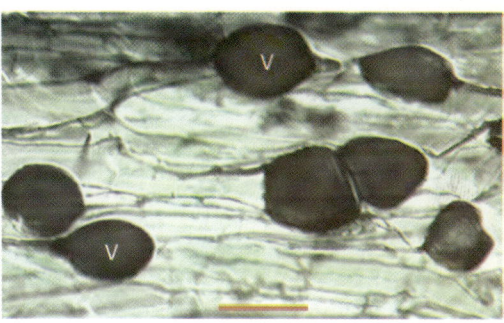

Fig. 1.3: Vesicles

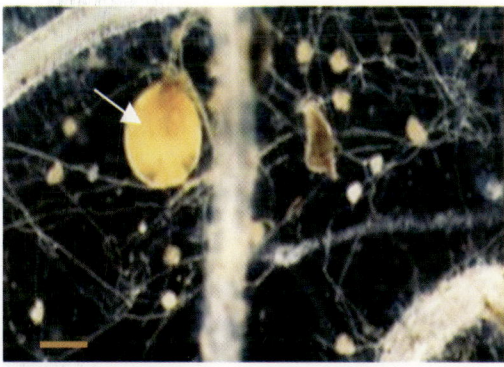

Fig. 1.4: VAM showing fine roots with root hairs

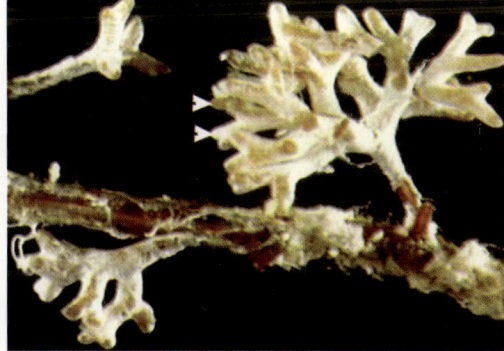

Fig. 1.5: Showing dichotomously branched roots of *Pinus* sp. with ectotrophic fungal mantle around roots

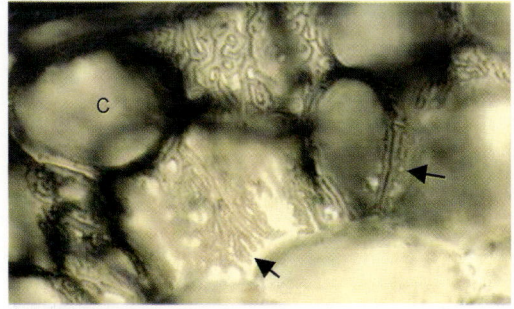

Fig. 1.6: Showing site of nutrient transfer

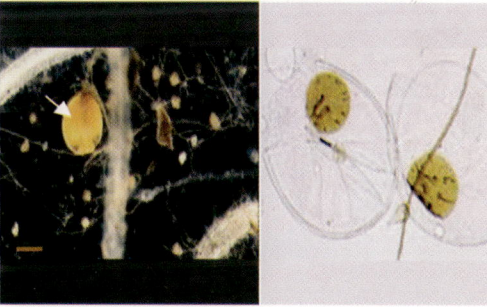

Fig. 1.9: *Gigaspora* and *scutellospora*

Plate 2

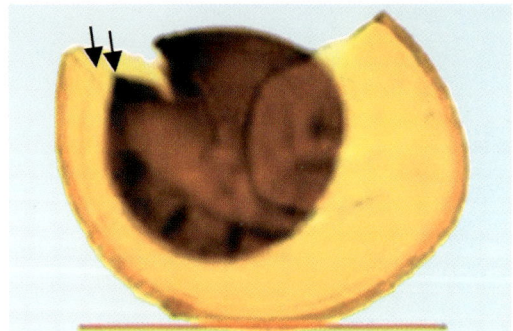

Fig. 1.10: Sporiferous saccule

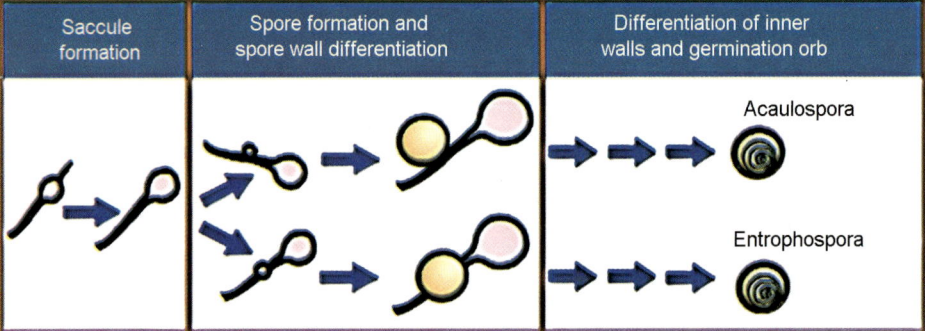

Fig. 1.11: Showing saccule formation

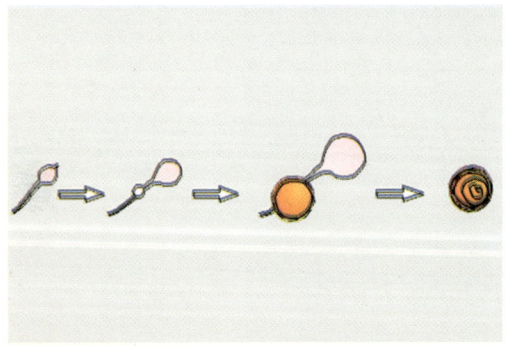

Fig. 1.12: Showing spore development in *Entrophospora*

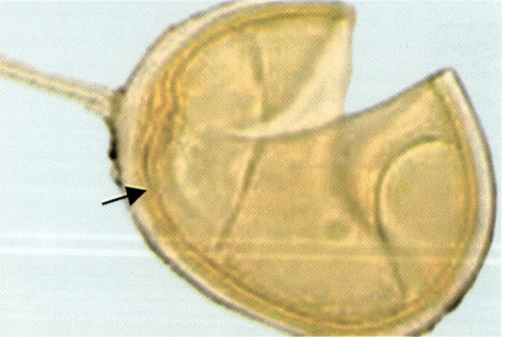

Fig. 1.13: *Glomus*

Plate 3

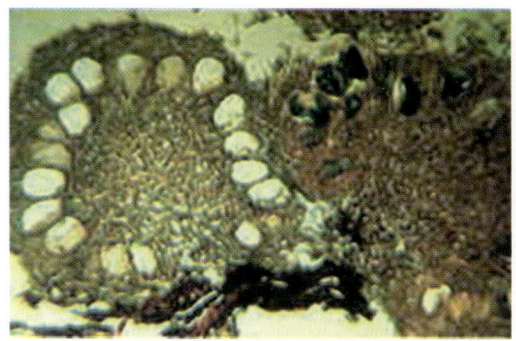

Fig. 1.14: *Sclerocystis*

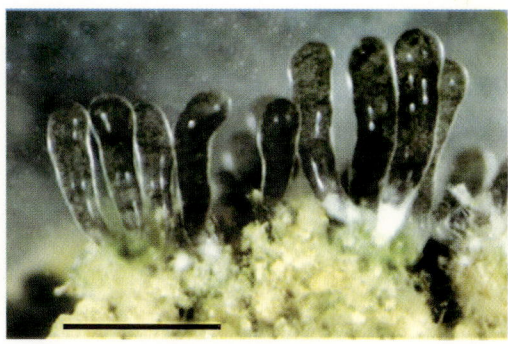

Fig. 1.15: *Geosiphon*

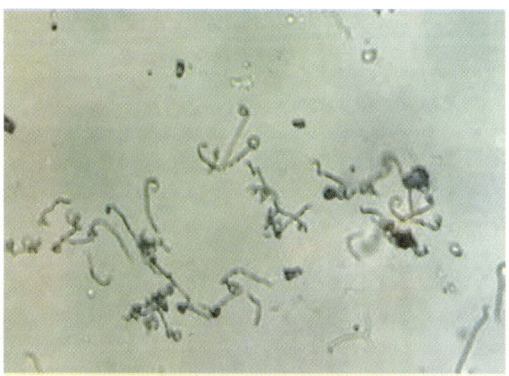

Fig. 5.1: Spiral spore chains (400 X)

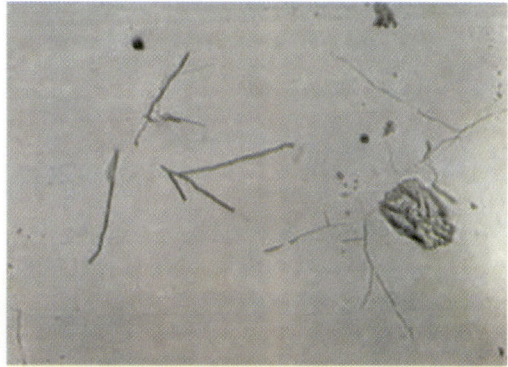

Fig. 5.2: RF spore chains (400 X)

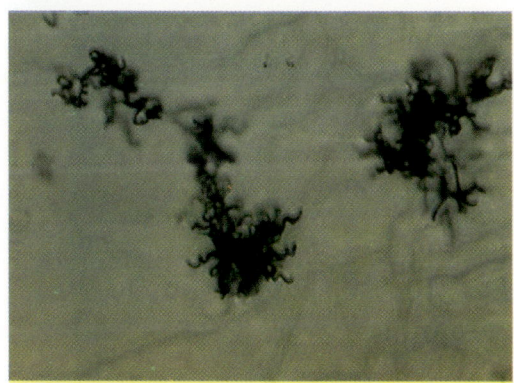

Fig. 5.3: RA spore chains (400 X)

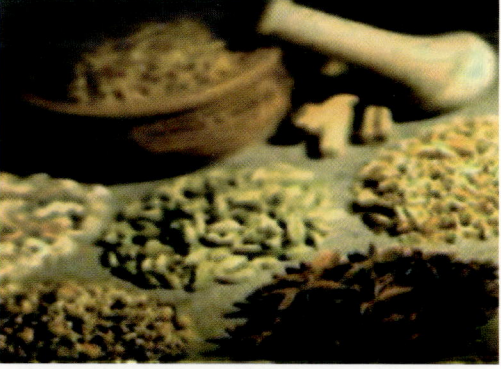

Fig. 6.1: Different spices used as alternative medicine throughout the world

Plate 4

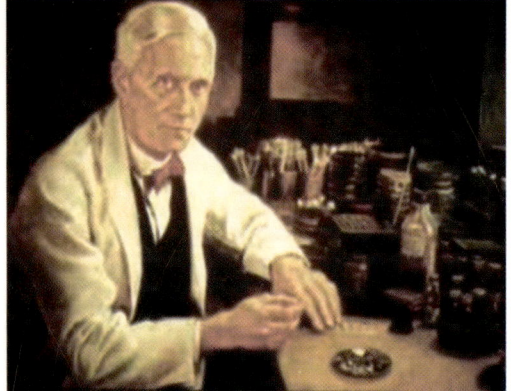

Fig. 6.2: Alexander Fleming, working in his laboratory

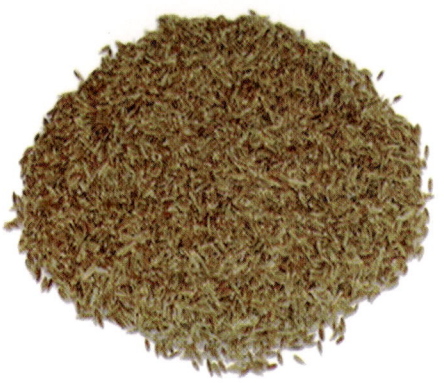

Fig. 6.3: Cumin seeds

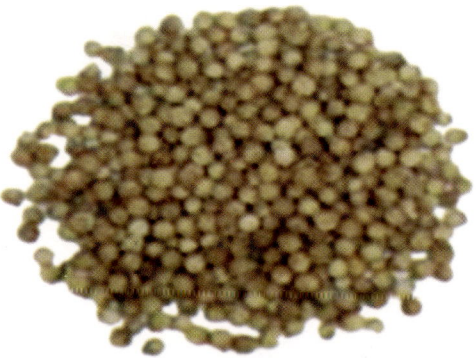

Fig. 6.4: Coriander seeds

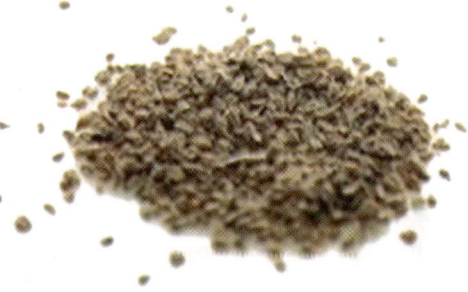

Fig. 6.5: Azwain seeds

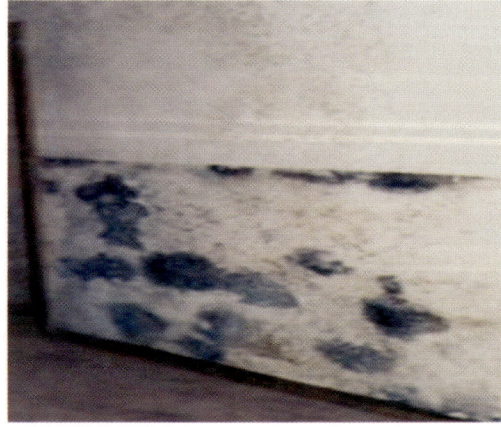

Fig. 9.1: Building deteriorating fungi

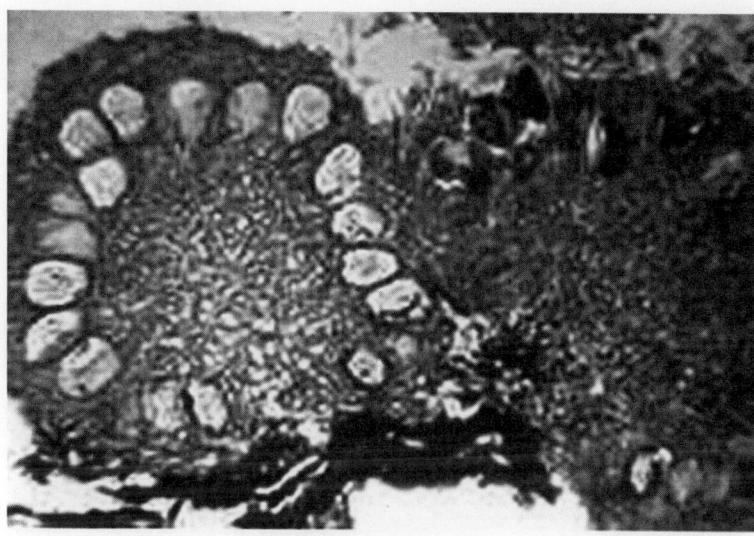

Fig. 1.14: *Sclerocystis*

Mycorrhizae are present in 92% of plant families (80% of species), with arbuscular mycorrhizae being the ancestral and predominant form, and indeed the most prevalent symbiotic association found in all the plant kingdom. The structure of arbuscular mycorrhizae has been highly conserved since their first appearance in the fossil record, with both the development of ectomycorrhizae, and the loss of mycorrhizae, evolving convergently on multiple occasions (wikipedia).

Vesicular-arbuscular Mycorrhizae and their Role in Biotechnology

The diagnostic feature of arbuscular mycorrhizae (AM) is the development of a highly branched arbuscule within root cortical cells. The fungus initially grows between cortical cells, but soon penetrates the host cell wall and grows within the cell. Vesicular-arbuscular mycorrhizae (VAM) are mutualistic symbioses formed between the roots of most plants and fungi in the order Glomales. The Glomales are currently classified in the Zygomycetes. Recent information from sequences of their 18S ribosomal genes indicates that they form an ancient group branching before the Ascomycetes and the Basidiomycetes (Rosendahl and Dodd, 1995). Vesicular-arbuscular (VA) and arbuscular mycorrhizae are endomycorrhizae formed by Zygomycete-like fungi and the roots of most families of Angiosperms as well as Gymnosperms, Pteridophytes and Bryophytes (liverworts). Non-mycotrophy in the angiosperms appears to be restricted primarily to the families Amaranthaceae, Brassicaceae, Chenopodiaceae and Zygophyllaceae, and many hemiparasitic plants. The mycorrhizal host may be facultatively or obligately dependent on its fungal partner. It appears that these mycorrhizal associations are evolutionary very old and that other types of mycorrhizae and non-mycotrophy evolved more recently. In fact, it has been speculated that VA mycorrhizae may have been involved in the successful invasion of land by vascular plants and played a controlling influence on the evolution of roots. Unlike many of the fungi involved in other types of mycorrhiza, these mycorrhizal fungi cannot be cultured in the absence of plant roots or a root organ culture.

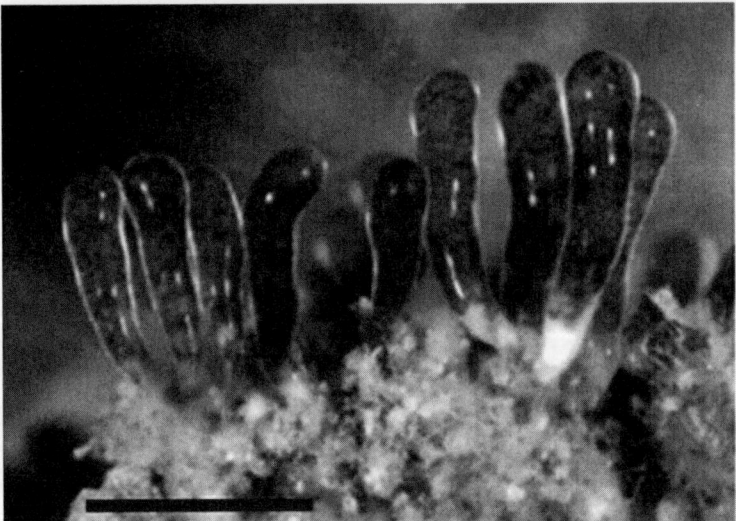

Fig. 1.15: *Geosiphon*

In contrast to most other types of mycorrhiza, the fungi do not substantially change the morphology of host roots. The presence of the fungi has to be determined by clearing, staining and microscopical examination of feeder roots. An experienced worker can readily recognise the coarse fungal hyphae with their distinctive angular morphology. These hyphae are restricted to the cortical region of the roots and never penetrate the stele. All the fungal species form arbuscules — small tree-like, hyphal-filled, invaginations of the cortical cells — which provide intimate contact between the plasmalemmae of the two symbiotic partners and are, presumably, the point of material exchange between host and fungus. They persist in active form for a very short period, 1 to 15 days. With the exception of species of *Gigaspora* and *Scutellospora*, the fungi form vesicles within the roots. These are lipid-filled, terminal swellings of hyphae with a storage/perennating function.

That members of two genera do not form vesicles has led to a debate as to whether the name arbuscular mycorrhizae is more appropriate than vesicular-arbuscular mycorrhizae for this relationship or whether the more appropriate of the two terms should be used depending on the fungal species present.

A 5 cm segment of living root can be colonised by as many as eight species from three genera of VA mycorrhizal fungi (Tommerup, 1988) and a germinated spore can simultaneously colonise roots of unrelated plants. Tommerup (1988) reported hyphae from a single spore of *Glomus caledonium* (Nicol and Gerd), Trappe and Gerd colonising roots of lettuce (*Lactuca sativa* L. - Asteraceae), white clover (*Trifolium repens* L. - Fabaceae) and rye grass (*Lolium perenne* L. - Poaceae) with living mycelium interconnecting at least one intraradical colony in each plant. There is considerable evidence that the mycorrhizal fungi enhance phosphorus uptake of their host plants and that their presence is more prevalent in roots in low P soils. These mycorrhizae also increase the uptake of other mineral nutrients. According to Sieverding (1991), for P, Cu and Zn, the VA fungi may act similarly to fertilization but that this is not the case for Fe. Mycorrhiza formation has also been shown to confer drought and disease resistance, reduce pest damage and nematode infection, promote seed production, and increase the fitness of plant offspring.

The AM type of symbiosis is very common as the fungi involved can colonize a vast taxonomic range of both herbaceous and woody plants, indicating a general lack of host specificity among this type. However, it is important to distinguish between specificity, innate ability to colonize, infectiveness, amount of colonization, and effectiveness, plant response to colonization. AM fungi differ widely in the level of colonization they produce in a root system and in their impact on nutrient uptake and plant growth (Fox, 1990).

The term biotechnology has been used for last two decades, major advances have generated new set of tools, which allow exploiting the biological resources much more meaningful. These tools of modern biology represent an integration of advances and techniques that fall largely in the areas of different fields such as biotechnology, cellular biology, molecular biology, genetics and microbiology. One such biological tool that is now being integrated into biotechnology is the development of AM inoculants for use in agriculture, horticulture, forestry and environmental reclamation. Basic studies have demonstrated that mycorrhizal associations play an important part in plant nutrition. The plants colonized by AM fungi harbour greater amount of phosphorus and other trace elements, specially when these are sparingly soluble (Abbott and Robson, 1984). AM infected plants also exhibit improved resistance towards drought, environmental stress and some root pathogens.

Ericaceous Mycorrhizae

The term ericaceous is applied to mycorrhizal associations found on plants in the order Ericales. The hyphae in the root can penetrate cortical cells (endomycorrhizal habit); however, no arbuscules are formed. Three major forms of ericaceous mycorrhiza have been described:

1. *Ericoid:* Cells of the inner cortex become packed with fungal hyphae. A loose welt of hyphae grows over the root surface, but a true mantle is not formed. The ericoid mycorrhizae are found on plants such as *Calluna* (heather), *Rhododendron* (azaleas and rhododendrons) and *Vaccinium* (blueberries) that have very fine root systems and typically grow in acid, peaty soils. The fungi involved are *Ascomycetes* of the genus *Hymenoscyphus*.

2. *Arbutoid:* Characteristics of both EM and endomycorrhizae are found. Intracellular penetration can occur, a mantle forms, and a Hartig net is present. These associations are found on Arbutus (e.g. Pacific madrone), *Arctostaphylos* (e.g. bearberry), and several species of the *Pyrolaceae*. The fungi involved in the association are *Basidiomycetes* and may be the same fungi that colonize EM tree hosts in the same region.

3. *Monotropoid:* The fungi colonize achlorophyllous (lacking chlorophyll) plants in Monotropaceae (e.g. Indian pipe), producing the Hartig net and mantle. The same fungi also form EM associations with trees and thereby form a link through which carbon and other nutrients can flow from the autotrophic host plant to the heterotrophic, parasitic plant.

Orchidaceous Mycorrhizae

Mycorrhizal fungi have a unique role in the life cycle of plants in the *Orchidaceae*. Orchids typically have very small seeds with little nutrient reserve. The plant becomes colonized shortly after germination, and the mycorrhizal fungus supplies carbon and vitamins to the developing embryo. For *Achlorophyllous* species, the plant depends on the fungal partner to supply carbon throughout its life. The fungus grows into the plant cell, invaginating the cell membrane and forming hyphal coils within the cell. These coils are active for only a few days, after which they lose turgor and degenerate and the nutrient contents are absorbed by the developing orchid. The fungi participating in the symbiosis are *Basidiomycetes* similar to those involved in decaying wood (e.g. Coriolus, Fomes, Marasmus) and pathogenesis (e.g. *Armillaria* and *Rhizoctonia*). In mature orchids, mycorrhizae also have roles in nutrient uptake and translocation.

Mixed Infections

Several fungi can colonize the roots of a single plant, but the type of mycorrhiza formed is usually uniform for a host. In some cases, however, a host can support more than one type of mycorrhizal association. Alnus (alders), Salix (willows), Populus (poplars), and Eucalyptus can have both AM and EM associations on the same plant. Some ericoid plants have occasional EM and AM colonization.

An intermediate mycorrhizal type can be found on coniferous and deciduous hosts in nurseries and burned forest sites. The ectendomycorrhiza type forms a typical EM structure, except the mantle is thin or lacking and hyphae in the Hartig net may penetrate root cortical cells. The ectendomycorrhiza is replaced by EM as the seedling matures. The fungi involved in the association were initially designated "E-strain" but were later shown to be ascomycetes and placed in the genus *Wilcoxina*.

Mechanisms of VAM

The mechanisms of VAM influence are still quite applicable (e.g. Safir et al, 1972; Reid, 1979). Perhaps because of the difficulty in consistently evoking or detecting VAM effects on host water balance, we have not improved our mechanistic understanding much in the intervening years. Further, in water relations work, cause and effect can be difficult to distinguish, which adds some ambiguity and overlap to the following discussion.

The best understood "mechanism" of VAM influence on host water balance involves VAM effects on plant size. The size of a plant can affect its water relations and drought responses and VAM symbiosis often affects plant size. Enhanced P acquisition is the most dramatic means by which VAM fungi affect overall plant biomass, but VAM effects on carbon and nitrogen relations and possibly other aspects of host biochemistry can also influence host size. VAM symbiosis also frequently changes the relative allocation of biomass within the plant. Both overall plant size and within-plant relationships, such as root-to-shoot ratios, can influence plant behavior, particularly when soil water becomes limiting.

Total Biomass

Other things being equal, more water usually moves in the soil-plant-air continuum per unit time through large plants than small plants. When VAM plants have different soil drying or gas exchange rates than smaller NM plants, this is often similar to NM plants having different soil drying or gas exchange rates than smaller NM plants. VAM-induced changes in total plant size probably affect plant water relations and drought responses mostly through effects on tissue hydration: How quickly tissues lose water and how quickly they can replace it?

Obviously, whole-plant transpiration rates will be higher in large than in small plants, even when transpiration rates per unit leaf area are equal. VAM plants constrained to the same soil volumes as smaller NM plants can thus be expected to deplete the available soil water more quickly than NM plants, eventually resulting in relatively lower tissue hydration and slowed foliar gas exchange in VAM plants. In experiments comparing VAM plants to smaller NM plants in relatively unrestricted soil volumes, e.g. experiments in the field or in large, non-root bound pots, the reverse may occur. Drought-induced tissue dehydration may be allayed in VAM plants having deeper or more extensive root systems.

Within-plant Size Relationships

VAM colonization can change specific root length, root architecture and root/shoot ratio (e.g. Berta et al., 1993). Consequently, even in VAM and NM plants having similar shoot dry weights and leaf areas, differing ratios of root length/leaf area might alter shoot response to soil drying. When a relatively larger, more finely divided or more efficient root system improves access to soil water and enhances leaf hydration, the cascade of associated responses is likely to be affected: Biophysical responses such as stomatal conductance, transpiration and to some extent photosynthesis, and biochemical responses such as compatible and total solute accumulation, enzyme activities, etc. It is often taken for granted that the root mass available for water absorption and supply to any given leaf area probably affects the rate of water loss by that leaf area, when soil moisture is limiting. Examination of stomatal responses of the cowpea cultivar used by Augé et al. (1992 a), however, revealed no dependence of stomatal conductance upon leaf area/root mass ratio. Others have also failed to detect a relationship between shoot/root ratio and rate of water loss per unit leaf area (Eavis and Taylor, 1979), although such relationships can occur (Meinzer et al., 1991). It has been suggested that extraradical hyphae may enhance the ratio of below-ground absorptive surface to leaf surface. Significant water uptake and transport by hyphae have been observed or computed in instances in which the VAM symbiosis has also affected stomatal behavior (Allen, 1982; Faber et al., 1991; Ruiz-Lozano and Azcón, 1995). When VAM-induced changes in stomatal conductance or transpiration of the host have been absent, hyphal contributions to water uptake have been negligible (Graham and Syvertsen, 1984; Fitter, 1985; George et al. 1992; Koide, 1993; Tarafdar, 1995). Not all VAM-induced developmental changes that might affect water balance need do so by affecting tissue hydration. For instance, root/shoot ratios can affect stomatal conductance directly, even in amply watered soils in the absence of effects on leaf hydration (Meinzer et al., 1991). Within-plant size relationships may also influence stomatal behavior by affecting hormone relations and concentrations of xylem constituents. VAM symbiosis may alter host water relations wherever plant size and development rates affect water relations. Although simple and perhaps physiologically prosaic, this influence probably has profound ecological and agricultural consequences, by affecting plant establishment, vigor, productivity and survival in water-limiting conditions (Robert, 2001).

Beneficial Effects of AM Result from One or Several of Mechanisms

a. Increased overall absorption capacity of roots due to morphological and physiological changes in the plant. There is increased absorption surface area, greater soil area explored (since the fungus acts as an extension of the root), greater longevity of absorbing roots, better utilization of low-availability nutrients, and better retention/storage of soluble nutrients, thus reducing reaction with soil colloids or leaching losses.

b. Increased mobilization and transfer of nutrients (P, N, S, micronutrients Cu, Zn) from the soil to the plant. Mycorrhizal fungi have been estimated to "substitute" up to 500 lb/a of P for citrus and 170 lb/a for soybeans in tropical areas.

c. Better development of P solubilizing bacteria in the mycorhizosphere.

d. Increased establishment, nodulation and atmospheric nitrogen fixation capacity in legumes.

e. Modification of plant-pathogen relations: Mycorrhizae influence the colonization of roots by other microorganisms, reduce the susceptibility (or increase the tolerance) of roots to soil-borne pathogens such as nematodes or phytopathogenic fungi such as *Fusarium oxysporum, Fusarium solani, Rhizoctonia solani* and *Macrophomina phaseolina*. Usually, plants of soybeans, cotton, tomato, oats, and cucumbers are less susceptible to nematode invasion, when they are mycorrhizal. In studies with fungi such as *Pythium, Phytophthora, Fusarium* and *Verticillium*, in most cases (53%) the mycorrhizal interaction is beneficial for onions, cucumbers, and tomatoes.

f. Secretion of antibiotics and support of a community that competes or antagonizes pathogenic microorganisms, thus aiding in disease suppression.

g. Increased production of plant growth hormones such as cytokinins and gibberelins.

h. Modification of soil-plant-water relations, promoting better adaptation of plant to adverse environment conditions (drought, metals). At elevated heavy metal concentrations in soils, mycorrhizal fungi have been shown to detoxify the environment for plant growth (Muchovej, 2001).

ROLE OF MICROORGANISMS IN MYCORRHIZAL FUNGI

Beneficial Microorganisms

In the great majority of natural communities, the primary producers depend heavily on microorganisms. Some of the microbes are symbionts, as in the case of mycorrhizae and nitrogen fixers. Others are free-living, but nevertheless linked tightly to the well-being of the primary producers. These include the organisms that decompose and mineralize organic detritus, others that promote plant growth and suppress plant pathogens, and some that build soil structure. There is considerable overlap between some of these groups. Plant species that are highly dependent upon mycorrhizae or other microbes have been difficult to work with during and after the nursery stage, because the symbionts are lacking on site or suppressed by horticultural practices. Intentional introduction of the beneficial microorganisms sometimes makes the difficult plant species easier to grow. The use of these organisms is not yet a turnkey operation. The importance of the beneficial microorganisms is in ecosystem functionality. These organisms help the roots take up nutrients, bring nutrient elements into the ecosystem from atmospheric or mineral reserves, breakdown detritus, release mineral elements in soluble form, and protect the roots from pathogens. They also hold soil aggregates together, creating channels through which roots grow, soil animal move, and water percolates. This assumes great importance, when we wish to produce a functional ecosystem on a previously disturbed site. A functional ecosystem, with its defining properties of sustainability, resistance to invasion, productivity, nutrient retention, and biotic interactions (Ewel, 1987), is a product of photosynthesis and all the microbial processes. To establish these processes, all organisms must be present and conditions must be compatible with their needs. Few of the organisms, and none of the functions, are present at severely disturbed planting sites. Unlike pathogens and opportunistic fungi, the important organisms do a poor job of dispersing. If we do not assure their presence and functionality, there will be no ecosystem. The kinds of organisms we will consider are mycorrhizae, nitrogen fixers, decomposers, plant growth promoting rhizobacteria, pathogen suppressive microorganisms, soil structure-building organisms, and cryptogamic crust organisms. The kinds of micro-organisms are beneficial to mycorrhiza fungi and many other organisms (Ted, 1992).

Vesicular-arbuscular Mycorrhiza (VAM): A Potential Biofertilizer

Vesicular-arbuscular mycorrhiza (VAM) is the most abundant kind of mycorrhiza described as 'a universal plant symbiosis'. They are found in practically every taxonomic group of plants and the list of species not infected is probably far shorter than the infected ones. Lack of host specificity is even more characteristic of this symbiosis than other types known. Studies on VAM fungi conducted during last few decades envisaged their occurrence in a wide variety of hosts, different habitats and variability in quality and quantity. Widespread distribution both in terms of habitats and host species, symbiotic relationships since the advent of terrestrialization, host growth promotiveness and protection, obligate nature and non-specificity for host, positive interaction with other rhizosphere microbes and several other characteristics of VAM fungi have obviously forced to find out their practical aspects. After the development of isolation techniques, mass production methods and inoculation, VAM fungi have been regarded as a boon for agriculture, forestry and restoration of disturbed ecosystems. The needs for indigenous VAM species isolation, screening and identification have been emphasized for these purposes. It has been a common experience that although chemical fertilizers have doubled the agricultural productivity but the mycorrhizal infection together with spore production have decreased. There is a need to use the VAM fungi as biofertilizers together with the minimum use of other chemicals. Experiments as done in agriculture have also been considered for trees and other plants for forest development. Although a few studies have been conducted on tropical trees, the results are encouraging as the growth of seedlings and productivity was found to be enhanced. The use of VAM fungi in forestry appears to be more important than in agriculture because in countries like India no large scale provisions exist to irrigate, fertilize and protect the plantation. The practical use of VAM fungi seems to be more appropriate as they are effective in overcoming the stress conditions like draught, disease incidences and deficiency of nutrients.

Application of Mycorrhizae in Agriculture

Ectomycorrhizal inoculum is easily produced for application in forest nurseries, but the necessity of AM inoculum production via a host plant is still an obstacle to ample utilization of AM fungi in agricultural crops. Nevertheless, progress is being made in this area and some commercial inoculum is currently marketed in the US. Some of the important practical applications of mycorrhizae are in soil/substrates (including transplanting media) that are constantly fumigated or receiving high rates of fungicides to eliminate/reduce soil-borne pathogens. With increasing concerns about excessive nutrient application to the environment, the use of mycorrhizal symbioses to promote plant growth while reducing the inputs of fertilizer and pesticides may have great potential for citrus and vegetable crops, which respond very well to inoculation (Muchovej, 2001).

VAM Fungi, Pollutants, Herbicides and Pesticides

Work with AMF strains tolerant to heavy-metal has provided evidence for their rapid adaptation to contaminated soils. Joner and Leyval (1997) found that cadmium-tolerant *Glomus mosseae* isolates AMF were responsible for uptake, transport and imobilization of cadmium. Copper (Cu) was absorbed and accumulated in the extraradical mycelium of three AMF isolates, as observed in a study with *Glomus* sp. (Gonzalez-Chávez et al. 2002). Other references indicated resistance of arbuscular mycorrhizal fungi to aluminum. Soil aluminum normally causes significant reduction in tissue calcium and magnesium concentrations (Cumming and Ning, 2003).

Glomus caledonicum seems to be a promising mycorrhizal fungus for bioremediation of heavy metal contaminated soil (Liao et al., 2003). Rufykiri et al. (2002) found that AM fungus could uptake and translocate uranium towards the roots. At varying zinc levels, mycorrhizal colonization increases zinc absorption and accumulation in the roots. This may help to explain the alleviation of zinc toxicity at high concentrations (Chen et al. 2003). Mycorrhizae were found to ameliorate the toxicity of trace metals in polluted soils growing in soybean and lentil plants (Jamal et al. 2002). In *Cynara cardunculus* mycorrhiza survived to pesticide employed in commercial nursery and enhanced wild carrdoon plant productivity (Marin et al. 2002).

Mycorrhizal colonization, however, was reduced in field plots through applications of the fungicide benomyl as a soil drenches (O'Connor et al. 2002).

Restoration of Degradated Areas Using VAM Fungi

The soils of disturbed sites are frequently low in available nutrients and lack the nitrogen-fixing bacteria and mycorrhizal fungi usually associated with root rhizospheres (Cooke and Lefor, 1990). As such, land restoration in semi-arid areas faces a number of constrains related to soil degradation and water shortage (Whisenant, 1999; Valejo et al., 2002a, b). As mycorrhizae may enhance the ability of the plant to scope with water stress situations associated to nutrient deficiency and drought, mycorrhizal inoculation with suitable fungi has been proposed as a promising tool for improving restoration sucess in semi-arid degraded areas (Pigott, 1982). By stimulating the development of beneficial microorganisms in the rhizosphere (Pennington, 1986), the use of VAM-infected plants could reduce the amount of fertilizer needed for the establishment of vegetation and could also increase the rate at which the desired vegetation becomes established by stimulating the development of beneficial microorganisms in the rhizosphere (Pennington, 1986). Degraded soils are common targets of revegetation efforts in the tropics, but they often exhibit low densities of AMF fungi (Michelsen and Rosendahl, 1990). This may limit the degree of mycorrhizal colonization in transplanted seedlings and consequently hamper their seedling establishment and growth in those areas. Soil inoculation with *G. mosseae* has significantly enhanced plant growth and biomass production in limestone mine spoils (Rao and Tak, 2002).

Root Pathogens

The phenomenon of AMF protecting plants from root pathogens is known from studies involving root-infecting pathogens, e.g. *Phytophthora parasitica* or *Fusarium* sp. root-invading nematodes (Dodd, 2000) and horticulutural and agricultural species such as tomato (Lycopersicum esculentum Mill.), alfalfa (Medicago sativa L.) (Dehne and Schonebeck, 1979), and in grasses (Newsham et al., 1995). *G. mosseae* induced local and systemic resistance to *P. parasitica* and was effective in reducing symptoms produced by this pathogen (Pozo et al., 2002). Larsen and Bodker (2001), however, found that in severely infected root cortical tissue *Glomus mosseae* had reduced energy reserves and biomass and did not protect the plant from the biotrophic pathogen, *Aphanomyces euteiches*. In wheat, high levels of colonization by AMF did not protect crop roots from damage by root pathogens (Ryan et al. 2002).

Plant Diversity and Soil Aggregation

Van der Heidjen et al. (1998) have provided evidence that diversity of AMF determines plant community structure through the response of individual plant species to this diversity. AMF diversity is the major factor in the maintenance of plant biodiversity and ecosystem stability and function. Several studies show that AMF alters plant community structure by affecting the relative abundance of plant species and plant-species diversity (Grimme et al. 1987; Gange et al. 1990; Sanders and Koide 1994). Interplant transport of assimilates from the dominant canopy species via a common mycorrhizal network to subordinate plant species, has been suggested as a mechanism by which AMF affect the floristic diversity of plant communities (Grimme et al. 1987). Another mechanism by which AMF may affect plant community structure is the differential growth response of plant species to colonization by AMF, the so-called "mycorrhizal dependence" (Gederman, 1975; Plenchete et al., 1983; Habate and Manjunath, 1991). The species composition and diversity of AMF communities has the potential to determine plant population and plant community structure. The fact that plant species vary in the degree of response to AMF species has important implications for growth of individual plant species. In turn, this will affect a plant's ability to coexist with other plant species in a community (Van der Heijden et al.,

1998). On the other hand, established mycorrhizal plants may serve as important sources of inoculum for initially nonmycorrhizal, conspecifics, which may affect regeneration and could contribute to patchy distributions of species within the community (Koide and Dickie, 2002).

VAM MANAGEMENT AND PERSPECTIVES

The main areas in which the benefits of introducing inoculant AMF into a plant growth system will accrue, are those in which they are lacking indigenous inoculum of AMF. These include sterilised soils or post *in vitro* plant micropropagation, buried, extremely fertilised, degraded areas (Dodd, 2000) or rooting of pepper cuttings (Thanuja et al., 2002). It is widely accepted that plants with highly branched root system (Gramineae) are less mycotrophic (less dependent on the fungi for normal Quilambo 543 growth) than those with coarser roots (e.g. cassava, onion). Root branching determines plant dependence on the symbiosis. Soils under low-input management show higher VAM fungus spore populations than soils under conventional management (Galvez et al. 2001; Douds et al., 1993, 1995). Early colonizing sand dunes species are nonmycorrhizal, whereas the later seral grasses are colonized with AMF.

Survival of AMF in soil may be affected by the presence or absence of crops and by the crop being grown (Troeh et al. 2003). The same author also reported differences related to crop succession. Fallow on fields had less spores than cultivation of corn followed by soybean, independently of the cultivars of corn or soybean. In cowpeas, inoculation and amendment with organic manure resulted in increased growth and yield. Inoculation with AMF and addition of composted grape pomace was beneficial to plants. This has been interpreted as the result of mycorrhizal fungus enhancing P uptake through extraradical hyphae. Such uptake increases nutrient use efficiency (Linderman and Davis, 2002).

In some cases, composted municipal waste addition and mycorrhizal inoculation were effective tools in programmes for revegetation of shrub species in semiarid mediteranean. The use of native mycorrhizal as a potential source of AM inoculum was considered a preferential strategy for ensuring the successful re-establishment of native shrub species in semi-arid degraded soil (Caravaca et al. 2003 b). Bell et al. (2003) found that the susceptibility of Acacia seedlings to colonization by AMF appeared to be seasonal. Colonization increased with increasing daytime temperatures and daylength. Despite the beneficial effects of AMF, their activity may be greatly limited by soil fumigation, non-responsive plant varieties, or rotations based primarily on non-mycorrhizal crops or crops of low AMF dependency. Salicylic acid contents in the plant reduced mycorrhization, suggesting that enhanced salicylic acid levels in plants delay AMF root colonisation. Although salicylic acid affects AMF root colonization, it has no effect on the potential of plants to be colonized by AMF (Medina et al., 2003). Manipulation of agricultural systems to favour AMF colonization must occur only if there is clear evidence that AMF make a positive contribution to yield or are vital for maintenance of ecosystem health and sustainability (Ryan et al., 2002).

Mycorrhizal Diversity is Important

Natural areas generally contain an array of mycorrhizal fungal species. The proportions and abundance of mycorrhizal species often shifts following any disturbance. Not all mycorrhizal fungi have the same capacities and tolerances. Some are better at imparting drought resistance while others may be more effective in protecting against pathogens or have more tolerance to soil temperature extremes. Because of the wide variety of soil, climatic, and biotic conditions characterizing man-made environments, it is improbable that a single mycorrhizal fungus could benefit all host species and adapt to all conditions. For example, the types and activities of mycorrhizal fungi associated with young plants may be quite different from those associated with mature plants. Likewise, mycorrhizal fungi needed to help seedlings establish themselves on difficult sites may differ from those which sustain productivity over a long-lived plant.

Diversity likely provides a buffering capacity not found on sites with only one or few species. The diversity of mycorrhizal fungi formed by a given plant may increase its ability to occupy diverse below-ground niches and survive a range of chemical and physical conditions (Amaranthus, 1999).

REFERENCES

1. Abbott LK, Roboson AD 1984. The effect of mycorrhiza on plant growth., in VA mycorrhiza. pp 113–130 ed CL powell and DJ Bagyaraj (USA: CRC Press, boca Raton, FL).

2. Amaranthus MP, Trapee JM 1993. Effects of erosion on Ecto-and VA-mycorrhizal inoculum potential of soil following forest fire in Southwest Oregon. *Plant* and *Soil*, (150): 41–49.

3. Anderson RC, Liberta AE 1989. Growth of little bluestem (Schizachyrium scoparium) (Poaceae) in fumigated and nonfumigated soils under various inorganic nutrient conditions. *American Journal of Botany* 76:95–104.

4. Ames RN, Reid CPP, Porter L, et al. 1983. Hyphal uptake and transport of nitrogen from two 15N-labelled sourcesby Glomus mosseae, a vesicular-arbuscular mycorrhizal fungus. *New Phytol.* 95:381–396.

5. Ahmad N. 1996. An assessment and enumeration of vesicular-arbuscular mycorrhizal propagules in some forest soils of Jengka. *Journal of Tropical Forest Science* 9:137–146.

6. Allen MF 1991. *The Ecology of Mycorrhizae*. Cambridge L'nlversity Press. New York.

7. Akond MA, Mubassara S, Rahman MM, Alam. S and Z.U.M. khan 2008. Status of vesicular-arbuscular (VA) mycorrhizae in vegetable crop plants of Bangladesh. *World Journal of Agricultural Sciences* 4 (6): 704–708.

8. Akond, M.A. and Z.U.M. Khan, 2001. Vesicular-arbuscular mycorrhizal fungi in timber yielding plants of Bangladesh. *Bangladesh J. Microbiol.*, 18(2): 135–140.

9. Akond. M.A, Mubassara. S, Rahman. M.M, Alam.S and Z.U.M. khan 2008. Status of vesicular-arbuscular (VA) mycorrhizae in vegetable crop plants of Bangladesh. *World Journal of Agricultural Sciences* 4 (6): 704–708.

10. Blase Mafia, Nalini M. Nadkarnil, David P. Janos (1993). Vesicular-arbuscular mycorrhizae of epiphytic and terrestrial Piperaceae under field and greenhouse conditions Mycorrhiza No. 4 : 5–9.

11. Bell J; Wells S, Jasper DA, Abbott LK (2003). Field inoculation with arbuscular mycorrhizal fungi in rehabilitation of mine sites with native vegetation, including *Acacia* sp. *Aus. System. Bot.* 16(1): 131–138.

12. Caravaca F, Barea JM, Palenzuela J, Figueroa D, Alguacil MM, Roldan A (2003a). Establishment of shrub species in a degraded semiarid site after inoculation with native allocthhonous arbuscular mycorrhizal fungi. *Appl. Ecol.* 22(2): 103–111.

13. Chen BD, Li XL, Tao HQ, Christie P, Wong MH (2003). The role of arbuscular mycorrhiza in zinc uptake by red clover growing in calcareous soil spiked with various quantities of zinc. *Chemosphere* 50(6): 839–846.

14. Cooke JC, and Lefor MW (1990) Comparison of veiscular-arbuscular mycorrhizae in plants from disturbed and adjacent undisturbed regions of a costal salt marsh in Clinto, Connecticut, USA. *Environ. Manage.* 14 (1): 212–137.

15. Dodd JC (2000) The role of arbuscular mycorrhizal fungi in agro-and natural ecosystems. *Outlook on Agriculture* 29 (1):55–62.

16. Douds DD, Galvez L, Janke R, Wagoner P 1995 Effect of tillage and farming system upon populations and distribution of veisculararbuscular mycorrhizal fungi. *Agric. Ecosys. Environ.* 52:111–118.

17. Dehne HW, and Schonebeck F (1979). Untersuchungen zum einfluss der endotrophen mycorrhiza auf planzenkrankheiten. I. Ausbreitung von Fusarium oxysporum f. sp.lycopersici in tomaten. *Phyotologische Zeitshrift* 95:104–110.

18. Endomycorrhizal fungi in some Malaysian soils under 23. Jayaratne, A.H.R. and U.P. de Waidyanatha, 1982. No. 12: 328–359.

19. Fox,T.R., N.B. Comerford, and W.W. McFee. 1990. Kinetics of phosphorus release from spodosols: Effects of oxalate and formate. *Soil Sci. Soc. Am. J.* 54:1441–1447.

20. Grimme JP, Mackey ML, Hillier SA and Read DJ (1987). Floristic diversity in a model system using experimental micrososmos. *Nature* 328:420–422.

21. Gonzalez-Chavez C, D'Haen J, Vangronsveld J, Dodd JC.2002. Copper sorption and accumulation by the extraradical mycelium of different Glomus spp (arbuscular mycorrhizal fungi) isolated from the same pol/ued soil. *Plant Soil* 240(2):287–297.

22. Gange AC, Brown VK and Farmer LM 1990. A test of mycorrhizal benefit in an early successional plant coumnity. *New Phytol.* 115:85–91.

23. Gederman JW 1975. Vesicular-arbuscular mycorrhizae.pp 575–591. In: J.C. Torey and D.P Clarkson (eds). *The Development and Function of Roots.* Academic Press, NY, USA.

24. Habate M and Manjunath A 1991. Categories of vesicular-arbuscular mycorrhizal dependency of host species. Mycorrhiza 1:3–12.

25. Harrison MJ. 2005. "Signaling in the arbuscular mycorrhizal symbiosis". *Annu Rev Microbiol.* 59: 19–42.

26. Joner EJ and levylal C. 1997. Uptake of roots by roots and hyphae of glomus mosseae/koide RT, Dickie IA. 2002. Effects of mycorrhizal fungi on plant populations. *Plant Soil* 244 (1–2): 307–317.

27. Liao JP, Lin XG, Cao ZH, Shi YQ, Wong MH .2003. Interactions between arbuscular mycorrhizae and heavy metals under sand culture experiment. *Chemosphere* 50 (6): 847–853.

28. Larsen J and Bodker L 2001. Interactions between pea rootimg-inhabiting fungi examined using signature fatty acids. *New Phytol.* 149:487–493.

29. Linderman RG and Davis EA 2002. Vesicular-arbuscular mycorrhiza and plant growth response to soil amendment with composed grape pomace or its water extract. *Phyton-Annales Botanicae* 11(3): 446–450.

30. Medina MJH, Gagnon H, Piche Y, Ocampo JA, Garrido JMG and Vierheilig H 2003. Root colonization by arbuscular mycorrhizal fungi is affected by the salicyclic acid content of the plant. *Plant Sci.* 164(6). 993–998.

31. Marin M, Ybarra M, Fe A and Garcia-Ferriz L (2002). Effect of arbuscular mycorrhizal fungi and pesticides on Cyanara cardunculatus growth. *Agricultural and Food Science in Finland 11* (3): 245–251.

32. Michelsen A and Rosendhal S (1990). The effect of VA mycorrhizal fungi, phosphorus and drought stress on the growth of Acacia nilotica and Leucaena leucocephala seedlings. *Plant Soil* 133:79–83.

33. M. Sharif and 2A.M. Moawad, 2006. Arbuscular Mycorrhizal Incidence and Infectivity of Crops in North West Frontier Province of Pakistan. *World Journal of Agricultural Sciences* 2 (2): 123–132.

34. Newsham KK, Fitter AH and Watkison AR (1995). Arbuscular mycorrhiza protect an annual grass from root pathogenic fungi in the field. *J. Ecol.* 83:991–1000.

35. O'Connor PJ, Smith SE and Smith EA .2002. Arbuscular mycorrhizas influence plant diversity and community structure in semi-arid herbland. *New Phytol.* 154 (1): 209–218.

36. Orlando António Quilambo., 2003. The vesicular-arbuscular mycorrhizal symbiosis. *African Journal of Biotechnology* Vol. 2 (12): 539–546.

37. Plenchette CA, Fortin A and Forlan N 1983. Growth response of several plant species to mycorrhiza in a soil of moderate P-fertility. I. Mycorrhizae aunder field conditions. *Plant Soil* 70:199–203.

38. Pennington JC 1986 Feasibility of using mycorrhizal fungi for enhancement of plant establishment on degraded material disposal sites; A literarature review. Miscellaneous Paper D-86–3. US Army Engineer Waterways Experiment Station, Vicksburg, Mississipi, USA.

39. Pigott CD 1982. Survival of mycorrhizas formed by Centroccocumgeophilum in dry soils. *New Phytol.* 92:513–517.

40. Pozo MJ, Cordier C and Dumas-Gaudot E 2002. Localized versus systemic effect of arbuscular mycorrhiszal fungi on defence responses to Phytophthora infection in tomato plants. *J. Exp. Bot.* 53(368): 525–534.

41. Robert. M. Auge. 2001. Water relations, drought and versicular Arbuscular mycohrriza. *Spinger link.* 11: 3–42.

42. Rufykiri G, Thiry Y, Wang L, Delvaux B and Declerck S 2002. Uranium uptake and translocation by the arbuscular fungus, Glomus intraradices, under root-organ culture conditions. *New Phytol.* 156 (2): 275–281.

43. Rao AV and Tak R 2002. Growth of different tree species and their nutrient uptake in limestone mine spoil as influenced by arbuscular mycorrhizal (AM)-fungi in Indian arid zone. *J. Arid Environ.* 51 (1): 113–119.

44. Ryan MH, Norton RM, Kirkegaard JA, McCormick KM, Knights SE and Angus JF (2002). Increasing mycorrhizal colonisation does not improve growth and nutrition of wheat on vertsols in south-eastern Australia. *J. Agric. Res.* 53 (10): 1173–1181.

45. Sanders IR and Koide RT 1994. Nutrient acquisition and community structure in co-occuring mycortrophic and non-mycotrophic old-field annuals. *Funct. Ecol.* 8: 77–84.

46. Trifolium subterraneum mycorrhiza from soil with high and low concentrations of cadmium. *New Phytol.* 135:53–360.

47. Thanuja TV, Hedge RV and Sreenivasa MN (2002). Induction of rooting and root growth in black pepper cuttings (Piper nigrum L.) with inoculatioon of arbuscular mycorrhizae. *Scientia Horticulture.* 92 (3–4): 339–346.

48. Troeh ZI and Loynachan TE (2003). Endomycorrhizal fungal survival in continuous corn, soybean and fallow. *Agron. J.* 95(1):224–230.

49. Tommerup, I.C. (1988) The vesicular-arbuscular mycorrhizas. *Advances in Plant Pathology* 6:81–91.

50. Turk, M.A., T.A. Assaf, K.M. Hameed and A.M. Al-Tawaha, 2006. Significance of Mycorrhizae. *World J Agri Sci* 2 (1): 16–20.

51. Vallejo VR, Serrasloses I, Cortina J, Seva JP, Valdecantos A and Vilagrosa A. (2000b). Restoration strategies and actions in Mediterranean degraded lands. In: Enne, G, Zanolla Ch, Peter D. (eds). *Desertification in Europe: Mitigation Strategies, Land use Planning*, Oofice for Official Publications of the European Communities, Luxembourg, pp. 221–233.

52. Van der Heijden MGA, Boller T, Wiemken A and Sanders JA 1998 Different arbuscular mycorrhizal fungal species are potential determinats of plant community strucuture. *Ecology* 79 (6) : 2082–2091.

53. Whisenant SG 1999. *Repairing Damaged Wildlands.* Cambridge University Press, Cambridge, p. 312.

2

Symbiotic Nitrogen Fixation and its Application in Microbial Biotechnology

Deepti Soni • Leena Parihar

NITROGEN FIXATION: AN INTRODUCTION

In atmosphere, there is about 80% of molecular nitrogen (N_2) which cannot be directly utilized as nitrogen fertilizer by plants. So this is a great irony of the botanical world. Nitrogen is an essential nutrient present in plant and it is required for plants, animals and human life.

The nitrogen is present in the atmosphere in the form of inert gas. This nitrogen cannot be utilized directly by higher plants. The higher plants assimilate only fixed forms of nitrogen like as nitrate ammonium ions. The nitrogen reacts with certain elements or compounds under suitable conditions to form fixed form of nitrogen, then the process is referred to as **nitrogen fixation**. So the nitrogen fixation can be defined as the conversion of free nitrogen into nitrogenous salts to make it available for absorption by plants.

In leguminous crops, legumes are rich in protein and it constitutes the very important role in human and animal nutrition. The symbiotic relationship between a bacterium called *Rhizobium* and legumes can provide large amounts of nitrogen to the plant and subsequently to soils where they are grown. In this process, the bacteria form nodules on the root system and convert the nitrogen that is coming from air into ammonia.

In this, the fixed nitrogen is required that biosynthesize the basic building block of life, e.g. amino acids for proteins and nucleotides for DNA. So this is a very essential process in life. Nitrogen fixation is utilized by numerous prokaryotes (aerobic bacteria, anaerobic bacteria and actinobacteria). Those microorganisms that fix nitrogen are called as diazotrophs. But some of the higher plants and animals like as termites also showed the symbiotic association with diazotrophs.

Manian *et al.* (1984) studied the nitrogen fixation and carbon dioxide assimilation in *Rhizobium japonicum* cultures. In free living cultures of *Rhizobium japonicum*, the

27

stimulatory effect of carbon dioxide on nitrogenase was mediated by ribulose bisphosphate carboxylase activity and this activity could be detected by using strains. The mutant strains show the pleiotrophic effects on carbon metabolism and they also possess the reduced level of hydrogen uptake, formate dehydrogenase, and phosphoribulokinase activities. Carbon dioxide is also helpful to promote vegetative growth and is also used to regulate the important cellular process like as hydrogen metabolism and nitrogen fixation. So due to this, it is helpful to increase the symbiotic association.

Hristozkova *et al.* (2009) investigated the growth and nitrogen fixation of different *Medicago sativa, Sinorhizobium meliloti* associations under conditions of mineral elements shortage. *Sinorhizobium meliloti* is a α-proteobacterium that alternates between a free-living form in soil and a symbiotic association within the nodules of host plant cells, where the nitrogen is fixed by bacteria ultimately differentiate into nitrogen-fixing organelle-like cells, called bacteroids and then released to plants in exchange for photosynthesis. Rhizobia developed specific genetic mechanisms to sense in the soil and *in planta*, then respond to various stresses, like as nitrogen and carbon starvation, oxygen limitation, etc. (Sauviac *et al.* 2007) So this study was designed to compare the difference in responses to nitrogen and carbon limitation in free living *Sinorhizobium meliloti* strains and their ability to form symbiotic association with alfalfa (*Medicago sativa*) plants. Its affectivity was observed by the nodules forming in the roots. For this research, two mutants like *Sinorhizobium meliloti* NitR and *Sinorhizobium meliloti* TspO and a strain *Sinorhizobium meliloti* 1021 were used. These are helpful to study the general stress responses. In both starvation conditions, the most effective symbiotic system was established between alfalfa and *Sinorhizobium meliloti* TspO. It's having capacity to fix the nitrogen.

Nitrogen fixation is divided into two types:

1. Biological nitrogen fixation.
2. Non-biological nitrogen fixation (physical nitrogen fixation).

Biological Nitrogen Fixation

Biological nitrogen fixation was discovered by the Dutch microbiologist Marinus Beijerinck. The conversion of atmospheric nitrogen into inorganic or organic usable forms through the agency of living organisms is called as biological nitrogen fixation. It is a continuous cycle (Fig. 2.1) that is maintained by the decomposers and nitrogen bacteria. This process is carried out by two main types of microorganisms: those which are free living or asymbiotic and those which live in close symbiotic association with other plants. However, the third type of microbes that fixes nitrogen in association with the roots of grasses and cereals, is called as symbiotic nitrogen fixation.

In other words, we can say that the biological nitrogen fixation is a process that occurs when atmospheric nitrogen is converted into the ammonia by using enzymes (bacteria cease the enzyme production only in the presence of oxygen) and this is called as nitogenase. There are some basic requirements for nitrogen fixation:

1. Presence of enzymes nitrogenase and hydrogenase (present in bacteroids and other nitrogen fixing organisms).
2. A protective mechanism for the enzyme nitrogenase against O_2.
3. Electron carrier (non-heme iron protein).

4. Constant supply of ATP.

5. TPP, co-enzyme-A, inorganic phosphate and Mg^{++} as cofactors.

6. Presence of cobalt and molybdenum.

7. Carbon compound for trapping released as ammonia.

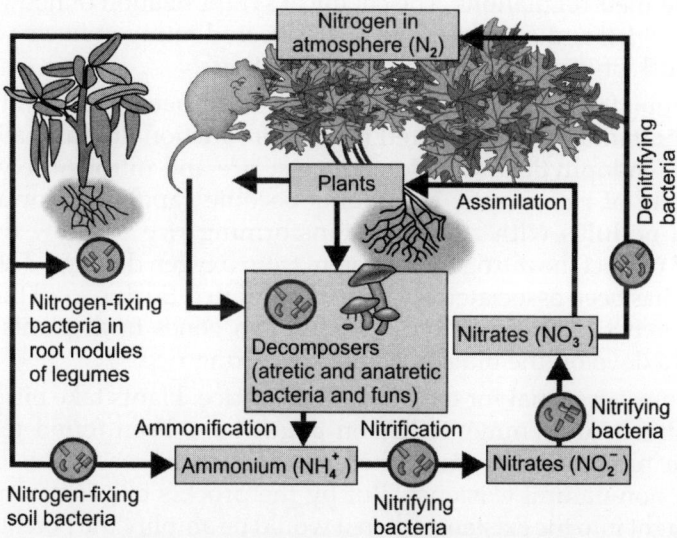

Fig. 2.1: Representation of nitrogen fixation cycle

In this, the non-heme iron protein (Fe) component reacts with ATP and reduces iron molybdenum protein (dinitrogenase), which then again reduces nitrogen to ammonia. The overall reaction of nitrogen fixation is as follows:

$$N_2 + 6\,H^+ + 6\,e^- \rightarrow 2\,NH_3$$

In this equation, it shows the reduction of nitrogen into ammonia and it is very energy intensive process. It requires at least 6 protons and 6 electrons. Besides this, it also requires at least 12 equivalent molecules of ATP (because 4 ATP are needed for each pair of electrons transferred to nitrogen). It is accompanied by the co-formation of one molecule of H_2.

After this the equation is modified as:

$$N_2 + 8\,H^+ + 8\,e^- \rightarrow 2\,NH_3 + H_2$$

This equation shows that an enzyme hydrogenase is present in almost all the microbes involved in N_2 fixation. Then after this, the enzyme catalyzes:

$$H_2 \rightarrow 2\,H^+ + 2\,e^-$$

In free-living diazotrophs, the nitrogenase-generated ammonium is assimilated into glutamate through the glutamine synthetase/glutamate synthase pathway.

Shihua and Yuxiang, (2003) collect the *Rhizobium* and developed the biological nitrogen fixation. They established the largest database of *Rhizobium* taxonomy and worked on the *Rhizobium* by different ways and presented work as international form.

They discovered the couple of *nif* genes, and then they found the regulative mechanism of positive regulation of *nif* genes and their sensitivity to oxygen, temperature. They also found the activity of nodulation gene *nod* D_3 product in *Sinorhizobium meliloti* (not controlled by flavonoid produced from its host alfalfa). They observed the association between expression of coding the products for carbon utilization and nitrogen metabolism and their regulations. The chemical synthesization of nodulation factor of *Sinorhizobium meliloti* and constructions of engineered nitrogen fixers were utilized in the research work of gene expression and regulation.

Sofi and Wani (2007) described the prospects of nitrogen fixation in rice. Nitrogen is the most important nutrient required for rice production. It is also a limiting factor. It improves the endophytic association between rice and nitrogen fixing bacteria. So after engineering of rice plants, rice plants become capable to form legumes like symbiosis and nodules with rhizobia, transforming rice to show the nitrogenase expression and protect the nitrogenase system from oxygen damage. The large number of diazotrophs has been associated with the roots of rice. So due to all these conditions, it will require genetic manipulation of nodulation genes from plants and *nif* genes from bacteria to develop the biological nitrogen fixing rice.

Nitrogen is most essential for the production of rice. Plants take nitrogen mostly in the form of nitrates and ammonia. Green plants have been found to be capable to obtain diatomic nitrogen from atmosphere. So due to this reason, biological nitrogen fixing rice is a non-natural existence. But by the process of genetic manipulation, if rice plants brought into the existence, then it would be amplify the potential for nitrogen supply and fixed nitrogen would be available directly to the plants without any loss. (Ladha and Reddy, 2000) That process was not very easy to done practically. It will require appropriate physiological conditions in the absence of environment that was normally provided by prokaryotic cell and it also require assembly of complex enzymes (Dixon *et al.*, 2000). This procedure was the challenge as well as the opportunity for the development and production of rice plants with inherent capacity to fix atmospheric nitrogen. If only half of the nitrogen applied to lowland, rice could be obtained from biologically fixed nitrogen, it would be save about 7.6 million tones of oil annually.

Examples of biological nitrogen fixing bacteria:

- Nitrogen fixation by non-leguminous plants
- Nitrogen fixation by *cyanobacteria*

Non-biological Nitrogen Fixation

Out of the total nitrogen fixation, 10% of nitrogen occurs by using physical process like lightning (i.e. electric discharge, thunder storms and atmospheric pollution). So nitrogen can be fixed artificially. This is a largest source of fixed nitrogen. In atmosphere, lightning and UV radiation favour for the combination of both gaseous nitrogen and oxygen then they form nitric oxide. Again nitric oxide becomes oxidized with oxygen and to form nitrogen dioxide.

The equation is as follows:

$$N_2 + O_2 \rightarrow 2\,NO \text{ (in the presence of lightning and thunder)}$$
$$2\,NO + O_2 \rightarrow 2\,NO_2$$

During rains, nitrogen dioxide combines with water and it forms nitrous acid and nitric acid. Then acids fall on the ground with rain water and react with alkaline radicals to produce water-soluble nitrates and nitrites.

$$2\ NO + H_2O \rightarrow HNO_2 + HNO_3$$

$$HNO_3 + Ca\ or\ K\ Salts \rightarrow Ca\ or\ K\ nitrates.$$

Then these nitrates are soluble in water and are directly absorbed by the plants.

The most common method of non-biological process is Haber process. This is largely energy-dependent process. In these days, nitrogen is manufactured by Haber-Bosch process (Burgess and Newton, 1977). This is very important process for nitrogen production. It requires high pressures (around 100–200 atm) and high temperatures (at least 400–600°C), for industrial catalysis. It uses natural gas as a hydrogen source and air as a nitrogen source, but for fertilizers petroleum is the main energy source (Ladha and Reddy, 2000). For global needs, fertilization production may also require fossil fuel energy that is equivalent to the 100 millions tones per year. Non-biological nitrogen fixation mostly used in fertilizers, explosives, etc.

Types of Nitrogen Fixation

There are three types of nitrogen fixation:
1. Symbiotic nitrogen fixation
2. Non-symbiotic nitrogen fixation
3. Associative nitrogen fixation

1. Symbiotic Nitrogen Fixation

The relationship between the plant and the bacteria is known as a symbiotic relationship or in other words we can say that all those association where two organisms live together symbiotically and the microbial partner fixes atmospheric nitrogen. The term symbiosis was coined by De Barry in 1879. In this, both the plant and the bacteria benefit from each other.

Many bacteria live symbiotically in the tissues of higher plants and perform nitrogen fixation. The best examples are found in bacterium *Rhizobium leguminosarum*, it belongs to family Leguminosae. Legumes including peas, lentils and alfalfa can form symbiotic associations for nitrogen fixation with a soil bacterium called *Rhizobium*. Rhizobia are Gram-negative, non-sporus, aerobic bacilli bacteria. The *Rhizobium* enters into the roots of plants and forms small tubercle-like structure called as root nodules (Fig. 2.2). The cells of root nodules then become quite large and polyploidy. Bacterial cells multiply rapidly inside these enlarged host cells and get transformed into somewhat swollen irregular forms called as bacteroides. They are founded in groups surrounded by the host membrane.

The cells of nodules present in the root tips contain a red or pink colour pigment called as leghaemoglobin. This pigment is distributed in the cytoplasm of the host cells and is a product of host tissue. Leghaemoglobin is similar to the haemoglobin of red blood cells and helps in the process of nitrogen fixation. It acts as oxygen scavenger, having ability to combine rapidly with oxygen and maintain the level of molecular oxygen low inside the nodules which activates the enzymes nitrogenase. Nitrogenase is an oxygen sensitive enzyme and it is active in anaerobic conditions. Rhizobia benefit

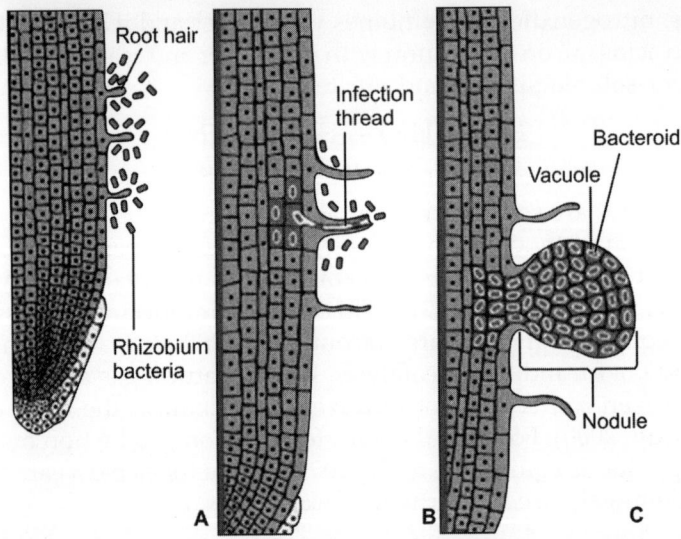

Fig. 2.2: Root nodules develop as a result of a symbiotic relationship between rhizobial bacteria and the root hairs of the plant. (A) The bacteria recognize the root hairs and begin to divide, (B) entering the root through an infection thread that allows bacteria to enter root cells, (C) which divide to form the nodule

as the plant provides carbohydrates (as a energy source). Carbohydrates are also produced by legume and transported to the root nodules of plants where they are used by the rhizobia as a source of hydrogen in the conversion of nitrogen to ammonia. So like this way, both the bacteria and roots are beneficial to each other. Rhizobia can also be added to soils through number of methods. It can be added by in furrow granule mix or by coated the seed with the bacterium (Fig. 2.3).

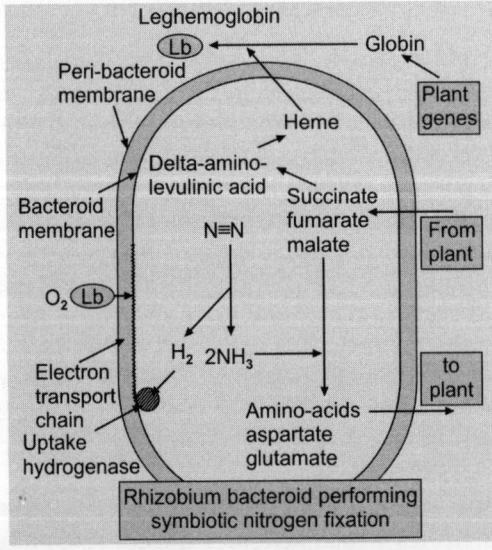

Fig. 2.3: Showing *Rhizobium* performing symbiotic N_2-fixation

Symbiotic nitrogen fixation is brought by certain bacteria, such as:

- *Rhizobium leguminosarum* (*Bacillus radicicola*) in the root nodules of legume.
- *Frankia* (of *Actinomycetes*) in the root nodules of *alnus, casuarina*, etc.
- *Klebsiella* in the leaf nodules of *dioscorrea*.
- *Rhizobium sebania* in the stem nodules of *Aeschynomene*.
- *Nostoc* and *Anabaena* (*Cyanobacteria*) in the coralloids roots of *cycas*.
- *Anabaena* as an endophyte in the leaf of *azolla*.
- *Nostoc* in the thallus of *anthoceros*.

There are a large number of examples where root nodules are not formed but symbiotic nitrogen fixation occurs. Some of the examples are given below:

1. *Lichens:* An association of fungi and algae (*Cyanobacteria* or *green algae*).
2. *Anthoceros* (a bryophyte) associated with *nostoc*.
3. *Azolla* (a fern) in association with *Anabaena azollae*.
4. *Cycas* coralloid roots in association with *Anabaena* or *Nostoc*.
5. *Gunnera macrophylla* (an angiosperm) stem in association with *Nostoc*.
6. *Paspalum notatum* (an angiosperm) roots in association with *Azotobacter* with *Azotobacter paspali*.
7. Roots of *digitaria, sorghum* and maize associated with *Spirillum notatum*.
8. Some nitrogen fixers grow on the surface of leaves of shrubs and trees. This was termed by Ruinen (1954) as "phyllosphere association".

Cocking *et al.* (1996) studied the symbiotic nitrogen fixation in cereals. They described about the interaction of rhizobia with cereals for nitrogen fixation. In symbiotic nitrogen fixation between soil bacteria and the member of plant family Leguminosae, rhizobia enter through the root hairs or by any cracks and cause infection. Then these form the morphological defined structure called as root nodules. Non-legume crops bring most of the significant contribution in biotechnology. Non-legume crops are known to be naturally forming nodules with either *Rhizobium* or *Bradyrhizobium parasponia* which are very closely associated to the growing tip of the roots by erosion of the surface of epidermal cells. Then it requires the initiation of cell division and followed by the formation of infection threads within the root cortex, after this cell division would occur and roots become swollen. The interaction of rhizobia with the root systems of cereals used to study whether an intracellular symbiotic nitrogen fixing association with rhizobia could be achieved of benefit to plant growth and development. In recent techniques, oxygen tolerant *Azorhizobium caulinodans* ORS 571 is isolated from stem nodules of the tropical legume *Sesbania rostrata* with the root systems of rice and wheat. The roots of both rice and wheat have been found the intracellular invasion of cells of the cortex in plants. By using acetylene reduction and 15 N dilution assays, these are active in nitrogen fixation. It helps to the beneficial growth.

Reid and Lloyd-Jones, (2009) described the nitrogen fixation in dampwood termite (*Stolotermes ruficeps*) in New Zealand. Termites thrive in tropical terrestrial ecosystems. It plays a very important role in the bio-recycling of lignocelluloses as the major decomposers of woody material. Due to the low nitrogen content of wood, a supply of usable nitrogen is essential for wood decomposition (Potrikus and Breznak, 1981). Reid and Gareth Lloyd-Jones described the diversity of nitrogen fixing organisms by using culture independent technique. Phylogenetic analysis of a portion of the *nifH* gene (encoding dinitrogenase reductase) revealed 19 phylotypes (>98% sequence identity) with 77–86% similarity to nucleotide sequences from uncultured microorganisms. From these studies, large number of sequences obtained were very closely related to sequences obtained from basal families Kalotermitidae, Termopsidae and the closely related wood-feeding cockroach species *Cryptocercus*. It indicates that the wood-dwelling termites are the important source of nitrogen into temperate forest. Large number of microorganisms living within the gut of termites and they consume wood material. So like this way, they are symbiont to each other. In this the nitrogen recycled again through proctodeal trophallaxis by dampwood termites (Machida *et al.* 2001).

2. Non-symbiotic Nitrogen Fixation

Soil contains a number of free living nitrogen fixing organisms. Most of these organisms live freely in soil or natural waters. These include a number of aerobic and anaerobic bacteria and blue green algae (e.g. *Cyanobacteria*). These are primitive nitrogen fixers. These organisms fix the nitrogen as ammonia actively under poor aeration by the reductional process. Nearly 40 species of blue green algae are known to fix nitrogen. These plants generally bear thick walled, hyaline heterocysts, which are the sites of nitrogen fixation.

The asymbiotic nitrogen fixers can be classified as follows:

1. *Free living aerobic nitrogen fixing bacteria: Azotobacter, Beijerinckia, Derxia.*
2. *Free living anaerobic nitrogen fixing bacteria: Clostridium pasteurianum, Bacillus.*
3. *Free living photosynthetic bacteria: Chlorobium, Rhodopseudomonas, Rhodospirellum.*
4. *Free living chemosynthetic bacteria: Desulfovibrio.*
5. *Free living fungi: Pullularia and yeasts.*
6. *Heterocyst bearing blue green algae (Cyanobacteria): Nostoc, Anabaena, Calothrix, Calothrix, Cylinderospermum, Tolypothrix, etc.*

Perez *et al.* (2003) described the non-symbiotic nitrogen fixation, net nitrogen mineralization and denitrification in five evergreen old growth forests and one second-growth forest of Chiloe Island, Chile: a comparison with other temperate forests. They studied about the biogeochemical cycles in the absence of industrial air pollution. By using acetylene reduction technique, non-symbiotic N fixation in the litter layer, mineral soil and coarse woody debris was estimated and by using buried bag method in the upper mineral soil layer, net-N mineralization was assessed. Denitrification rates of mineral soil were also assessed by the acetylene inhibition assay. In their results, the mineral soil of the northern temperate forests showed the highest N fixation rates. In the Chiloe forests, both the N mineralization and denitrification were lower as compared to the northern temperate forests. So due to this reason, southern temperate forests exert a stronger biotic control as compared to the northern temperate forests.

Holguin *et al.* (1992) investigated the two new nitrogen fixing bacteria from the rhizophore of mangrove trees and their isolation, identification and in vitro interaction with rhizosphere *Staphylococcus* sp. Mangroves are trees and shrubs which grow in the tidal zone of tropical and sub-tropical seas. (Clough, 1982) In this, the two new diazotrophic bacteria such as *Listonella anguillarum* and *Vibrio campbellii,* and one non-nitrogen-fixing bacterium, *Staphylococcus* sp. were isolated from the rhizosphere of mangrove trees. During purification, N_2-fixation of the bacterial mixtures becomes decreased but when these were grown in vitro in mixed cultures, then the nitrogen fixing capacity of *Staphylococcus* sp. becomes increased. It indicates that other species of rhizosphere bacteria, a part from the common diazotrophic species, should be evaluated for their contribution to the nitrogen-fixation process in mangrove communities; and the nitrogen-fixing activity detected in the rhizosphere of mangrove plants is probably not the result of individual nitrogen-fixing strains, but the sum of interactions between members of the rhizosphere community.

Atanassova: Altimirska and Bakalivanov (2009) described the gardian and pivot herbicide effect on some non-symbiotic nitrogen, fixing bacteria. In agriculture, the applications of herbicides can lead to soil pollution risk and may cause number of side effects on soil microflora. This is most important to investigate the impacts of herbicides for soil fertility and plant nutrition microorganisms. (Bakalivanov *et al.*, 1996 and Kruglov, 1991). Investigation of gardian and pivot effect was done by measuring the bacterial growth and free living non-symbiotic nitrogen-fixing bacteria such as *Azotobacter chroococcum* and the two strains of associative nitrogen fixer *Azospirillum brasilense* will give an information about the ecological assessment of these herbicides. Inhibition of bacterial growth is observed and it depends on the herbicide used, its concentration and the bacterial strain. At high concentration, gardian inhibition on the bacterial growth varies and the size of bacterial colonies becomes reduced and it showed that the gardian is more toxic than pivot as concerning the growth of the bacterial species.

3. Associative Symbiotic Nitrogen Fixation

Certain types of bacteria, living in close contact with the roots of cereals and grasses, fix nitrogen. This association is a loose mutualism, called as associative symbiosis nitrogen fixation. The bacteria reside in the transition zone between soils and root (the rhizophore) and sometimes enter the roots. Some of the fixed nitrogen is absorbed by the roots and in return the bacteria get nourishment from the carbohydrates released by the roots.

There are number of examples of associative nitrogen fixation:

1. *Azospirillum brasilense* in the association with cereal roots.
2. *Beijerinckia* in association with the roots of sugarcane.
3. *Azotobacter paspali* in associastion with roots of tropical grass — *Paspalum notatum*.

Besides the biological and non-biological nitrogen fixation, few other events can be discussed below:

1. Ammonification
2. Nitrification
3. Denitrification
4. Amino acid degradation
5. Proteolysis

Ammonification

It is a process of decomposition of nitrogenous organic compounds of the dead bodies of plants and animals into ammonia or ammonium or ammonium ions in the soil. It is carried out by some of the bacteria, e.g. *Clostridium, Pseudomonas, Bacillusramosus, Bacillus vulgaris* and *Bacillus mycoides*.

Ammonification can be carried out in two steps:

1. The proteins are broken down into their constituents amino acids.
2. Amino acid is transformed into ammonia. Some of the ammonia diffuses into the atmosphere. Ammonia as such toxic to the plants but ammonium ions can be safely absorbed by the plants. Therefore, ammonia does not remain in gaseous state in the soil but get changed into the ammonium ionic form.

Nitrification

It is a metabolic process by which ammonia is oxidized to nitrates through nitrites. This is brought by some nitrifying bacteria, e.g. *Nitrosomonas, Nitrosococcus* and *Nitrobacter*. It also involves two steps:

1. Ammonia is oxidized into nitrites. It is carried out by *Nitrosomonas* and *Nitrosococcus*.

$$2\ NH_3 + O_2 \rightarrow 2\ HNO_2 + 2\ H_2O + Energy$$
Nitrite bacteria

2. Nitrite is further oxidized to nitrate by *Nitrobacter*. Most of the nitrifying bacteria are chemoautotrophs. They use the energy liberated during nitrification.

$$HNO_2 + \tfrac{1}{2}\ O_2 \rightarrow HNO_3 + Energy$$
Nitrate bacteria

Denitrification

The nitrates and ammonia are converted to nitrous oxide and finally to nitrogen gas by several denitrifying bacteria, e.g. *Pseudomonas fluorescence, P. denitrification, Bacillus subtilis* and *Thiobacillus denitrification*.

$$6\ KNO_3 + 5\ S + 2\ H_2O \rightarrow K_2SO_4 + KHSO_4 + 3\ N_2 + energy$$
Thiobacillus

In this, the nitrogen gas is released from denitrification and it is lost to atmosphere. Then it completes the complex nitrogen cycle.

Amino Acid Degradation

It is carried out by many microorganisms which degrade amino acids to release ammonia.

$$Alanine + 1/2\ O_2 \rightarrow Pyruvic\ acid + NH_3$$
Alanine deaminase

Proteolysis

In this process, there is a breakdown of protein into simpler forms. It is carried out by number of microorganisms, e.g. *Clostridium, Pseudomonas, Proteus, Bacillus,* etc. It is also carried out by fungi. The microorganisms secrete extracellular enzymes, e.g. proteinases (which convert protein into the peptides) and peptidases (which convert peptides into amino acids).

Proteins $\rightarrow$ peptides $\rightarrow$ amino acid

Proteinases   Peptidases

ROLE OF BIOTECHNOLOGY IN SYMBIOTIC NITROGEN FIXATION

- In these days, biotechnology plays very important role for the symbiotic nitrogen fixation.
- It is very helpful in agricultures for the production of necessary things.
- It helps to improve the crop fertility.
- It helps to produce disease free varieties of plants. It can suppress the activity of pests and protect the plants.
- It helps to produce large varieties of plants even in desert conditions.
- It helps to save energy.

Abdel *et al.* (2004) described about the applications of microbial biotechnology for sustainable legume production in desert conditions. For future agricultural expansion in the Arab countries which are located in deserts, these applications gained experience by agricultural institutions for the production of necessary things such as food, feed and fibres. So due to these benefits in harsh conditions, dry environment will be turn into productive agricultural land. Legumes play a very important role in agriculture and these are very necessary for building the sustainable agricultural production systems. In desert agriculture, the legume-rhizobia biological nitrogen fixation (BNF) reduces the cost of production and preserves underground water from contamination with the excess nitrogen fertilizers required to insure the high productivity. Then the large amount of soluble nitrogen fertilizers could be leached with irrigation water and reaches the ground water. So due to the biological nitrogen fixation, this requirement is essential for growth of plant. They quantify the amount of nitrogen fixed by the peanut/*Rhizobium* symbiotic system in sandy soil. They revealed the application of rhizobial inoculants in the field through either injection with irrigation water, or as beat-based inoculant. But the native rhizobia were occupied 16 to 24% of nodules of the field-grown legumes by using fluorescent antibody (FA) technique. The efficiency of nitrogen fixation was determined by inoculant rhizobial strains and they also showed the presence of high numbers of native rhizobia in the soils.

Gurr *et al.* (2004) worked on the ecological engineering: A new direction for agricultural pest management. Odum (1962) was the first to use the term ecological engineering. Ecological engineering is considered for arthropod pest management approaches and contrasts with its controversial cousin genetic engineering. This requires the functional mechanisms that lead to components of biodiversity to suppress pest activity and exploited. Pest suppression via ecological engineering is placed in the broader context of ecosystem services provided by farm land biodiversity including nitrogen fixation and the conservation of pollinator species and wild life.

Parakaran (1997) described the benefits of biological nitrogen-fixing rice. There are number of benefits of biologically nitrogen-fixing rice plants to agriculture especially in poor developing areas.

- It helps to save energy. Plants require 16 ATPs for nitrogen fixation, which are much less than the Haber-Bosch process used for chemical fixation of nitrogen. Haber-Bosch process requires high temperature (400–600°C) and high pressure (100–200 atm). So due to this reason, it saves high energy inputs.

The equation of Haber–Bosch process:

$$N_2 + H_2 \rightarrow NH_4$$

- It also helps to save money (20 billion dollars) annually.
- Biological nitrogen fixing rice plants help to save environment. These are eco-friendly in nature. Carbon dioxide is released during chemical nitrogen fixation into the environment. So this causes global warming with severe implications and carbon dioxide is also a potential green house gas.
- It also helps to save labour. During the end of the season of rice growth, biological nitrogen fixing rice stubbles can be put into the soil that can act as a biofertilizers.
- It helps to produce large number of production of biologically nitrogen-fixing plants. Biologically, nitrogen-fixing plants have improved either their association with rhizobia or with *nif* genes and transfer then it has been found to be more productivity. This helps to improve the production of biologically nitrogen-fixing plants. In 2003, Papademerion showed the table and he compared the potential and feasibility of different kinds of systems in rice for the nitrogen fixation. Tables 2.1 and 2.2 represent the comparison between the conventional and free biological nitrogen fixation.

Table 2.1: Conventional biological nitrogen fixation system

Conventional BNF system	N_2-supply potential	Rice yield potential	Technology availability	Feasibility and adaptation
Fee living or associative	50–100 kg ha^{-1}	3.6 t ha^{-1}	3–5 years	High
Green manure	100–200 kg ha^{-1}	5–8 t ha^{-1}	Available	Low

Table 2.2: Free biological nitrogen fixation system

Free BNF system	N_2-supply potential	Rice yield potential	Technology availability	Feasibility and adaptation
Endophytic	?	?	3–5 years	High
Induced symbiosis	>200 kg ha^{-1}	>8 t ha^{-1}	>5 years	High
Nif genes transfer	>200 kg ha^{-1}	>8 t ha^{-1}	>5 years	High

BACTERIA RESPONSIBLE FOR NITROGEN FIXATION

All the nitrogen fixing organisms are prokaryotes (bacteria). Some of them live independently of other organisms, these are called as free living nitrogen-fixing bacteria. There are number of bacteria which are responsible for the nitrogen fixation:

- Diazotrophs
- Cyanobacteria
- Azotobacteraceae
- Rhizobia
- Frankia

Cyanobacteria play key roles in the carbon and nitrogen cycle of the biosphere. Generally, *Cyanobacteria* are able to utilize a variety of inorganic and organic sources of combined nitrogen, like nitrate, nitrite, ammonium, urea or some amino acids. Several *Cyanobacterial* strains are also capable of diazotrophic growth. *Calothrix, Cylinderospermum, Tolypothrix,* etc. are the examples *of Cyanobacteria. Cylinderospermum* is inoculated in the sugarcane and maize fields as nitrogen fixers.

Azotobacter species have the highest known rate of respiratory metabolism of any organism, so they might protect the enzyme by maintaining a very low level of oxygen in their cells. *Azotobacter* species also produce copious amounts of extracellular polysaccharide. Like this way, all other microorganisms are also responsible for nitrogen fixation.

Postgate (1970) studied the nitrogen fixation by sporulating sulphate-reducing bacteria including Rumen strains. For nitrogen fixation, acetylene test is important tool in reassessing the ability of various groups of microorganisms to fix nitrogen (Parejko and Wilson,1968; Millbank, 1969; Hill and Postgate, 1969). So after reassessment, it has been found that several types of aerobic genera such as *Azotomonas, Pseudomonas, Nocardia, Pullularia* and yeasts probably do not fix nitrogen, but the nitrogen fixation has been proved to be far more widespread among the sulphate-reducing bacteria of the genus *Desulfovibrio* than the earlier test which was studied by Reiderer-Henderson and Wilson, in 1970.

Apte and Prabhavathi (1994) investigated the rearrangements of nitrogen fixing genes in the heterocystous cyanobacteria. Cyanobacteria are also called as blue green algae and they are a fascinating group of photosynthetic bacteria that help to fix atmospheric nitrogen. In the vegetative cells of heterocystous cyanobacteria, such as *Anabaena*, two operons harbouring the *nif* genes contain two separate intervening DNA elements resulting in dispersion of genes and then impaired gene expression. It is of 11bp sequences that disrupt the *nif* D gene and it is directly repeated at its ends after this it harbours a gene. A large element of 55 kb interrupts the *fdx* N gene and at its end parts having 5 bp direct repeats. It accommodates at least one gene. During heterocystiscontis, both of the discontinuous excised by two distinct site specific recombination events. As consequences, both of the elements of 11 bp and 55bp are removed from the circles. Then it created the *nif* operons. After this in heterocysts, it expressed the nitrogenase protein from the rearranged genes and aerobic nitrogen fixation ensues.

Novel nitrogen-fixing *Acetobacter* species have been isolated from the semi-solid sugarcane juice and inoculated in medium with dilutions of 10^{-7} or 10^{-8} of sugarcane roots and stems. These showed higher nitrogenase activity (Lima *et al.*, 1987). They also suggested when *Acetobacter* colonies were grown in N-free semisolid sucrose medium then they will yield nitrogenase activity. But the nitrogenase activity can also be increased by increasing concentrations of yeast extract as 'N' source in the medium (Cavalcante and Dobereiner, 1988) and at low concentration when medium is complemented with NH_4Cl then it also showed the complete inhibition and repression of nitrogenase activity. The maximum nitrogen fixing activity showed by *Alcaligenes faecalis,* when it was demonstrated by You *et al.* (1991).

Keirn and Brezonik (1971) investigated the nitrogen fixation by bacteria in Lake Mize, Florida and in some lacustrine sediment. In these studies, they measured the nitrogen fixation in water column of Lake Mize, Florida by using acetylene reduction technique. But the results was showed for a very short period during summer stratification. From the water of Lake Mize, three bacterial cultures were isolated which are capable to fix nitrogen. But with the depth of 30–50 cm, cores rates become decreased and acetylene reduction was also detected in sediments of 7 out of 25 Florida lakes and in sediments from 3 Guatemala lakes, acetylene reduction occurred by the high concentrations of sucrose. It was not affected by any other materials. From these studies, they indicate that the bacterial fixation in aquatic environments is more widespread.

Gadgil and Bhide (1959) studied nitrogen fixation by *Azotobacter* in association with some associated soil microorganisms. This study was used to find out the effects of nitrogen fixation by *Azotobacter*, when it was grow in associations of four strains of *Azotobacter* (isolated from irrigated soils), number of soil microorganisms and *Actinomycetes* in mixed cultures in test tubes containing 10 ml of Ashby's manitol-phosphate dilution to which molybdenum, but iron was not added. After incubation period of 15 days, nitrogen was determined. Some of the strains of *Rhizobium* spp. and *Actinomycetes* stimulated nitrogen fixation greatly. So there is a possibility that legumes might have stimulatory effect on nitrogen fixation by *Azotobacter* cells, when it's having very close association with roots.

BIOTECHNOLOGY OF NITROGEN FIXATION AND *NIF* GENES

There are number of genes involved in nitrogen in plants and these genes are called as *nif* genes or fix genes. Mostly *nif* genes are found in free living nitrogen fixing bacteria and in symbiotic bacteria in various plants. They also include the structural genes for nitrogenase and other regulatory genes. *Nif* genes encode nitrogenase complex and other enzymes involved in nitrogen fixation. It has consenses sequences identical from one nitrogen bacteria to another, but the structure of the *nif* genes is similar and the regulation of the *nif* genes varies between different diazotrophes (=nitrogen fixing organisms). It depends upon organisms.

There are approximately 20 different *nif* genes that encode the nitrogenase complex. The *nif* (nitrogen fixation) proteins are often referred to by their gene names and their roles in nitrogen fixation.

nif J	= pyruvate flavodoxin reductase, involved in electrone transport to nitrogenase.
nif F	= flavodoxin
nif H	= dinitrogenase reductase obligate electrone donor to dinitrogenase during nitrogenase turnover. Also is reqired for FeMo-co biosynthesis and apodinitrogenase maturation.
nif M	= processing of maturation of *nif* H protein
nif K,D	= molybdoferredoxin
nif B,N,E,V,W,Z	= MoFe cofactor synthesis
nif Y	= MoFe cofactor insertion
nifQ	= molybdenum uptake
nif A,L,R	= regulation
nif U,S	= metal center biosynthesis
nif X,T	= function unknown (not necessary, at least under normal conditions)

The *nif* gene is the gene that is responsible for the coding of proteins related and associated with the fixation of atmospheric nitrogen into a form of nitrogen available to plants. Nitrogenase complex is the primary enzyme, which is composed of Fe (dinitrogenase) and Mo-Fe protein (dinitrogenase reductase), and it is encoded by *nif* genes, which is in charge of converting atmospheric nitrogen-N_2 to other nitrogen forms such as ammonia and these can be used by the plants for various purposes. The substantial molecular diversity of N_2 fixing bacteria has been detected in rice field. It is based on retrieval of *nif* H or *nif* D gene fragments from root DNA (da Rocha *et al.* 1986). Nitrogen fixing microorganism contains *nif* H genes, these were used to monitor the presence of these diazotrophs in pure cultures (Frank et al. 1998), in soil (Widmer *et al.* 1999) and plants and after this these were molecular characterize (on RAPD-PCR and rep-PCR) of their *nif* genes by using *nif* H primer (Berg *et al.* 1994). Besides the nitrogenase enzyme, the *nif* genes also encode a number of regulatory proteins involved in nitrogen fixation. The *nif* genes also showed the expression at low concentrations of fixed nitrogen and oxygen concentrations.

Palacios *et al.* (2005) studied the genetics and biotechnology of the hydrogen-uptake (NiFe) hydrogenase from *Rhizobium leguminosarum* bv. Viciae, a legume endosymbiotic bacterium. In this the frequent inhabitant of European soils becomes capable to establish the symbiotic association with peas, lentils, vetches and other legumes. In *R. leguminosarum* bv. Viciae, hydrogenase genes (*hupSLCDEFGHIJKhypABFCDEX*) are clustered in a 20 kbDNA region of the symbiotic plasmid. This plasmid also contains genes for nodulation and nitrogen fixation.

The location of hydrogenase genes in the symbiotic plasmid is a general trait for hydrogenase positive strains of *R. leguminosarum*, suggesting an adaptation of hydrogen recycling to the symbiotic lifestyle in this bacterial species (Leyva *et al.* 1990). Such adaptation is more evident, when looking at the regulation of the system. So the limited number of strains (that belong to the genera of Rhizobiaceae) was capable to express the hydrogenase system and nitrogenase evolved the partial or full recycling of hydrogen. So due to this reason, it increases the energy efficiency in nitrogen fixation process.

ENHANCEMENT OF BIOLOGICAL NITROGEN FIXATION

The process of biological nitrogen fixation has been researched for providing the efficient N inputs into plants since many years. It involves highly specialized and intricately evolved interactions between higher plants and soil microorganisms for harnessing the atmospheric elemental nitrogen (N). It has become abundantly clear that the host plant (legumes) dominates in regulating the biological nitrogen fixation process. This process is influenced by environmental factors. Perturbation or any manipulation of the interactions between the bacteria and the legumes seems to offset the critical balance, usually to the detriment of N fixation efficiency. But it has been unable to obtained more success either enhancing or transferring the traits of nitrogen fixation to non-nitrogen fixing organisms.

So for the improvement in agricultural traits, other alternative physiological approaches were used and these have been more successful as compared to non-biological nitrogen fixation. Then these are used for improving mobilization, redistribution and utilization of stored N reserves within the host plant.

Hamid *et al.* (2007) worked on the diagnosis of nutritional constraints of *Azolla* sp. that enhance their growth under flooded conditions of salt effected soils. *Azolla* is an aquatic pteridophyte that forms a regular permanent symbiosis, with a heterocysts forming nitrogen fixing, *Cyanobacterium*. A green housework was conducted to know the nutritional constraints of *Azolla* for enhancing its growth under flooded conditions. Then select the best ones for its use as biofertilizer in rice-wheat cropping system. From these tested nutrients (e.g. phosphorus, iron and zinc), phosphorus was found to be the major limiting nutrient for plant growth than other nutrients. *A. pinnata* var. *pinnata* and hybrid *Azolla Rong Ping* gave better growth hence can be used as biofertilizer in rice-wheat cropping system.

De Souza Moreira (2007) investigated diversity of soil: Genetic resources to enhance nitrogen fixation in agriculture and forestry. The soil diversity implies not only enhance, but also showed better knowledge for environment. Leguminosae is the third largest family of flowering plants. It was estimated around 2000 native species. From all of these, five native strains *Rhizobium tropici*, *Mesorhizobium plurifarium*, *Sinorhizobium adherens*, *Azorhizobium doebereinerae*, *Burkholderia mimosarum* were selected. This represents the important source for new species and strains of Leguminosae nodulating bacteria (LNB) to be explored and to enhance symbiotic nitrogen fixation. It has been represented the bacterial species/strains and plant species vary regarding the establishment of their symbiosis from highly specific, i.e. it was able to form symbiosis with just a narrow range of partner species/strains, to highly promiscuous. *Azorhizobium doebereinerae* and *Sesbania virgata* were highly efficient. Siratro (*Macroptilium atropurpureum*), common beans (*Phaseolus vulgaris*) and cowpea (*Vigna unguiculata*) are very well-known promiscuous hosts that established symbiosis with a large number of species and high nitrogen fixation efficiency. For the selection of strains and inoculants efficiency, specificity/promiscuity, efficiency and adaptability in environment conditions must be considered. Strain *M. loti* MAFF 303099 was the first LNB genome which was already sequenced and it involved symbiosis and nitrogen fixation when it was compared with other LNB genomes. Then he selected the efficient strains and used for inoculants production of 109 leguminous species. According to MAPA, in 2003, 99% of inoculants were produced, being for soybeans and remaining 1% for the other 108 species, these indices the diffusion of biotechnology and need to be improved. If inoculants were applied directly or indirectly to the other legume species then they showed benefits of nitrogen fixation that could enhance crop productivity in an environmentally sound way.

Verburg *et al.* (1979) studied about the non-symbiotic nitrogen fixation in 3-year-old Jeffrey pines and described the role of elevated (CO_2) of old Jeffrey pines. Non-symbiotic N_2 fixation could be stimulated under the elevated level of CO_2. So due to this, it helps to enhancing growth responses of vegetation to elevated CO_2 on nutrient-poor sites. This hypothesis can be tested by planting the non-symbiotic N_2 fixation rates in soils with 3-year-old Jeffrey pine. The rates of nitrogen fixation were estimated by measuring 15 N content of trees and soil. It was also compared with the ambient CO_2 treatment, so the elevated CO_2 treatment did not affect biomass, N content, or plant parts and soils. It indicates that it does not stimulate non-symbiotic N_2 fixation with elevated level of CO_2. Because belowground C inputs did not increase under elevated CO_2, the initial hypothesis could not be accepted or rejected. These studies showed that the non-symbiotic N_2 fixation is not likely to provide a large input of N in forest ecosystems and did not allow for firm conclusions to the effects by elevated level of CO_2.

REFERENCES

1. Abdel Al HM 2004. Application of Microbial Biotechnology for Sustainable Legume Production in Desert Conditions. *International Conf. on Water Resources and Arid Environment.*

2. Apte SK, Prabhavathi N. 1994 Rearrangements of nitrogen fixation (*nif*) genes in the heterocystous cyanobacteria *J. Biosc.*, 19: 579–602.

3. Atanassova – Altimirska R, Bakalivanov, D. 2009. Gardian and Pivot herbicide effect on some Non-Symbiotic Nitrogen Fixing Bacteria. *Institute of Soil Science, Sofia* 1080; 2009.

4. Bakalivanov D *et al.* 1996. Soil Science, *Agrochemistry and Ecology,* 3: 9–12.

5. Berg DE Akopyants NS, Kersulyte D. 1994. Fingerprinting microbial genomes using the RAPD or Rep-PCR method. *Methods Mol. Cellular Biol.,* 5: 13–24.

6. Burgess, B. K. And Newton, W. E. 1977. Nitrogen fixation . Its scope and importance. *Plew Press, New York, USA.*

7. Cavalcante, V. A. and Dobereiner, J. 1988. A new acid tolerant nitrogen fixing bacterium associated with sugarcane. *Plant Soil,* 108: 23–31.

8. Clough, B .F. 1982. In: Mangrove Ecosystems in Australia: structure, function and management, (Clough, B.F., Ed.), p. xv. *Colorcraft Ltd, Hong Kong.*

9. Cocking, E. C. Caroline A. Batchelor, C. A. Kothari, S. L., Jain, S., Webster, G. Jones, J., Jotham, J. and Davey, M. R. 1996. Cereal symbiotic nitrogen fixation–the interaction of rhizobia with cereals for symbiotic nitrogen fixation. *Plant Genetic Manipulation Group, University of Nottingham.*

10. Da Rocha, A., Okhi, S. T. and Hiuki, C. 1986. Detection of mycoplasma like organisms *in situ* by indirect by indirect immunofluorescense microscopy. *Phytopathology,* 76: 864–868.

11. De Souza Moreira, F. M. 2007. Soil biodiversity: genetic resources to enhance nitrogen Fixation in agriculture and forestry. *Lotus Newsletter Volume 37 (3): 112–113.*

12. Dixon, R., Cheng, Q. and Day. A. 2000. Prospects of constructing Nitrogen fixation cereals. In: The quest for Nitrogen Fixation in rice. Proc. 3rd working group meeting on assessing opportunities for Nitrogen fixation in rice. *IRRI. Los Banos, Phillipines, pp: 354.*

13. Frank, I. H., Fegan, M., Hayward, A. C. and Sly, L. 1998. Nucleotide sequence of the *nif* H gene coding for nitrogen reduction in the acetic acid bacterium *Acetobacter diazotrophicus. Lett.App.Microbiol.,* 26: 12–16.

14. Gurr, G. M., Wratten, S. D. and Altieri, M. A. 2004. Ecological engineering: a new direction for agricultural pest management. *AFBM Journal, 1:28–35.*

15. Gadgil, P. D. And Bhide, V. P. 1959. 1959. Nitrogen Fixation by *Azotobacter* in association with some associated soil microorganisms. *College of Agriculture Poona.*

16. Hamid, N., Sikander, A., Malik, K. A. and Hafeez, F. Y. 2007. Diagnosis of nutritional constraints of *Azolla* spp. to enhance their growth under flooded conditions of salt affected soils. *Pak. J. Bot., 39(1): 161–167.*

17. Hill, S. and Postgate J. R. 1969. Failure of putative nitrogen-fixing bacteria to fix nitrogen. *Journal of General Microbiology 5: 277–285.*

18. Holguin, G., Guzman, M. A. and Bashan, Y. 1992. Two new nitrogen-fixing bacteria from the rhizosphere of mangrove trees: Their isolation, identification and *in vitro* interaction with rhizosphere *Staphylococcus* sp. *FEMS Microbiology Ecology 101: 207–216.*

19. Hristozkova, M., Stancheva, I., Geneva, M. 2009. Growth and nitrogen fixation of different *Medicago sativa- Sinorhizobium meliloti* associations under conditions of mineral elements shortage . *Acad. M. Popov" Institute of Plant Physiology, Bulgarian Academy of Sciences.*

20. Keirn, M. A. and. Brezonik, P. L. 1971. Nitrogen fixation by bacteria in Lake Mize, Florida, and in some Lacustrine sediments. *University of Florida, Gainesville 3260l.*

21. Kruglov, J. V. 1991. Microflira and Pesticides, *Agropromizdat, Moskva, 122–129.*

22. Ladha, J. K. and Reddy, P. M. 2000. Steps towards Nitrogen fixation in rice. The quest for Nitrogen Fixation in rice. Proc. 3rd working group meeting on assessing opportunities for Nitrogen fixation in rice. *Los Banos, Phillipines, pp: 354.*

23. Leyva, A., Palacios, J. M., Murillo, J. and Ruiz – Argu eso, T. 1990. *J. Bacteriol. 172: 1647–1655.*

24. Lima, E., Boddey, B. M. and Dobereiner, J. 1987. Quantification of biological nitrogen fixation associated with sugarcane using a 15 N aided nitrogen balance. *Soil Biol. Biochem., 19:* 165–170.

25. Machida, M., Kitade O Miura, T., Matsumoto, T. 2001.Nitrogen recycling through proctodeal trophallaxis in the Japanese damp-wood termite *Hodotermopsis japonica* (Isoptera, Termopsidae). *Insectes Sociaux 48: 52–56.*

26. Manian, S. S., Gumbleton, R. ,Buckley, M. A.and Gara, O. F.1984. Nitrogen Fixation and Carbon Dioxide Assimilation in *Rhizobium japonicum. Applied and environmental microbiology, 48:* 276–279.

27. Millbank, J. W. 1969. Nitrogen fixation in moulds and yeasts-a reappraisal. *Archiv fur Mikrobiologie 68: 32–39.*

28. Parakaran, J. 1997. BNF rice: The choice of new generations. Paper presentation in plant genetic seminar on nitrogen fixation. *University of Wisconsin Madson Wisconsin, USA.*

29. Papademerion, M. K. 2003. Rice production in the Asia- Pacific region. Issues and prospective. *FAO document. FAO Rome. (www. FAO. Org/ DOCREP/ oo3/X 690SE/X 690SE/ X6905e 04. Htm)*

30. Parejkor, A. and Wilson, W. 1968. Taxonomy of Azotomonas species. *Journal of Bacteriologi, 95: 143–146.*3

31. Palacios, J. M., Manyani, H., Martinez M., Ureta, A. C., Brito B., Bascones, E., Rey, L., Imperial. J. Ruiz-Argueso, T. 2005. Genetics genetics and biotechnology of the H_2-uptake [NiFe] hydrogenase from *Rhizobium leguminosarum* bv. viciae, a legume endosymbiotic bacterium. *Biochemical Society Transactions Volume 33.*

32. Perez, C.A., Carmona, M. R., and Armesto, J. J. 2003. Non-symbiotic nitrogen fixation, net nitrogen mineralization and denitrification in evergreen forests of Chiloe island, Chile: a comparison with other temperate forests. *Gayana Bot. 60(1): 25–33.*

33. Postgate, J. R. 1970. Nitrogen Fixation by Sporulating Sulphate-reducing Bacteria Including Rumen Strains. *Journal of General Microbiology., 63: 137–139.*

34. Potrikus, C. J., Breznak, J. A. 1981. Gut bacteria recycle uric acid nitrogen in termites: a strategy for nutrient conservation. *Proceedings of the National Academy of Sciences, USA 78:* 4601"4605.

35. Reiderer-Henderson, M. A. and Wilson, P . W. 1970. Nitrogen fixation by sulphate-reducing bacteria. *Journal* of *General Microbiology 61: 27–32.*

36. Reid, M. N. and LLoyd-Jones, G.: Nitrogen Fixation in New Zealand dampwood termite. (*Stolotermes ruficeps*)2009. *New Zealand Journal of Ecology 33(1):* 90–95

37. Sauviac, L., Philippe, H., Phok, K., Bruand, C. 2007. *J Bacteriol, 189(11): 4204–4216.*

38. Shihua, S. and Yuxiang, J. 2003. Present status and development on biological nitrogen fixation research in China. *Chinese Science Bulletin 2003 Vol. 48(10): 954–960.*

39. Sofi, P. and Wani, S. 2007. Prospects of nitrogen fixation in rice. *Asian journal of plant sciences, 6(1): 203–213.*

40. Verburg, P. S. J., Cheng, W., Johnson, D. W. And Schorran D. E. 1979. Nonsymbiotic nitrogen fixation in 3-year-old Jeffrey pines and the role of elevated [CO2]. *Can. J. For. Res., 34.*

41. Widmer, F., Shaffer, B. T., Porteous, L. A. and Seidler, R. J. 1999. Analysis of *nif* H gene complexity in soil and litter at a Douglas fir forest site in the Oregan Cascade Mountain Range. *Appl. Environ. Microbiol., 65: 374–380.*

42. You, C. B., Song, N., Wang, H. X., Li, J. P., Lin, M. and Hai, W.L. 1991. Association of *Alcaligenes faecalis* with wetland rice. *Plant Soil., 137: 81–85.*

3

How Bacteria Communicate

Shailja Pant

Bacteria converse with one another and with plants and animals by emitting and reacting to chemical signals. The need to "talk" may help explain why the microbes synthesize a vast array of compounds.

Richard Losick and Dale Kaiser

All forms of communication between human beings have long been recognized as a requirement for reciprocal understanding, transfer of knowledge, and productive development of societies. This also applies to living cells that are organized in micro-societies that constantly adjust to their environment through a complex network of signaling pathways. The chemical communication which occurs at various levels results in an integrated exchange of information that is essential for coordinated responses (Perbal, 2003).

Several genetic and biochemical studies in 1960s and 1970s provide compelling evidences for an organized social behaviour employing sophisticated communication systems to coordinate the activities of individuals within a population. The concept that bacteria could talk to one another received attention only in 1980s. Such a system is accomplished by the extracellular accumulation of small, self-generated chemical signaling moieties that induce a concerted effort on behalf of a population to produce the desired phenotypic effect (Kievit and Iglweski, 2000).

Quorum Sensing

Quorum sensing is a bacterial cell to cell signaling system. The term quorum sensing was first used by Fuqua et al. (1994) for the process of chemical communication that bacteria use to assess cell population density and synchronize behaviour on a community-wide scale. The word *Quorum* means a fixed number of members of any body, society whose presence is necessary for the proper or valid transaction of business (Henderson et al. 2001). It is the regulation of gene expression in response to fluctuations in cell-population density. Quorum sensing bacteria produce and release chemical signal molecules called autoinducers that increase in concentration as a function of cell density. The detection of a minimal threshold stimulatory concentration of an autoinducer leads to an alteration in gene expression. Gram-positive and Gram-negative bacteria use quorum sensing communication circuits to regulate a diverse array of physiological activities. These processes include symbiosis, virulence, competence, conjugation, antibiotic production, motility, sporulation, and biofilm formation (Melissa et al. 2001).

Several classes of microbial-derived signaling molecules have now been identified. Broadly, these can be divided into two main categories (Dunny and Winans, 1999; Whitehead et al. 2001):

1. Amino acids and short peptide derivatives(commonly utilized by Gram-positive bacteria)
2. Fatty acid derivatives, called homoserine lactones, HSLs (commonly utilized by Gram-negative members)

Sporulation and fruiting body formation in *Myxococcus xanthus*, morphological differentiation in *Streptomyces coelicolor*, virulence mechanism of medically significant Gram-positive and Gram-negative bacteria, conjugation of *Enterococcus faecalis*, antibiotic production by *Streptomyces* sp. nitrogen fixing by *Rhizobium* sp. sporulation in *Bacillus subtilis* are some of the examples of cell-to-cell signalling.

Present understanding of quorum sensing is based on the discovery of luminescence produced by certain marine bacteria *Vibrio fischeri* and *Vibrio harveyi*. These bacteria form symbiotic relationships with some fishes such as *Monocentris japonica* (Japanese pinecone fish) and with species of squid *Euprymna scolopes* (bobtail squid). These marine animals contains very high population (10^{10}–10^{11} cells ml^{-1}) of a mono-specific culture of *V. fischeri* in their light organ due to which *E. scolopes* could express bioluminescence in dark environments (Visick and McFall-Nagai, 2000). The function of the light organ in the squid is due to the camouflaging behaviour called counter illumination. The squid camouflages itself from predators residing below it by controlling the intensity of light *via V. fischeri* that it projects downwards, thus eliminating a visible shadow created by moonlight. *E. scolopes*, in return, provides nutrients to the population of *V. fischeri*, thus a perfect symbiotic relationship. Sea water contains a large number of *Vibrio* species; however, this light organ appears to have a positive selection mechanism choosing only certain *V. fischeri* strains.

Bioluminescence

For a long time, bioluminescence expressed by *V. fischeri* remained a model system to study density-dependent expression of a gene function. The sudden increase in luminescence was attributed to the transcriptional regulation of the enzyme, luciferase, which in turn corresponded to a threshold density of cells (Hastings and Greenberg, 1999). This whole circuit is based on the bacterial assessment of its population density by means of chemical signaling molecules or autoinducers released by bacterial cells. The autoinducer then establishes a communication between the cells that gets reflected in the expression of a particular gene, in this case, the luciferase gene (*lux*). *Lux* system is an operon system involving two main regulatory genes and a number of other genes that synthesize the chemical reagents required to produce photons.

The first regulatory gene, i.e. *luxI* encodes a protein which catalyses the synthesis of the acyl homoserine lactone (AHL). This reaction uses S-adenosylmethionine as the donor of the homoserine lactone and a fatty acid moiety linked to an acyl carrier protein. The second regulatory gene, i.e. *luxR* encodes a protein which acts both as a receptor for AHL and as a transducer of the signal activating the other genes present in the lux operon. When AHL binds to the *luxR* protein the genes *lux-CDABEG* are expressed. The *luxA* and *luxB* genes encode the α and β subunits of bacterial luciferase. The other genes encode polypeptides that are involved in the synthesis of the substrate (tetradecanal) used by the luciferase to generate light (Henderson et al. 2001).

Molecular Basis of Bioluminescence Regulation

The bioluminescence gene cluster of *V. fischeri* consists of eight *lux* genes — *luxA-E, luxI* and *luxR,* which are arranged in two bi-directionally transcribed operons separated by about 218 bp (lux regulon) (Engerbrecht et al. 1983). One unit contains *luxR,* and the other unit, which is activated by the *luxR* protein along with the auto-inducer, contains the *luxCDABEG* operon. The products of both the *luxI* and *luxR* genes function as regulators of bioluminescence. The *luxI* gene is the only *V. fischeri* gene required for synthesis of the auto-inducer, 3-oxo-hexanoylhomoserine lactone (3-oxo-C6-HSL) or OOHL in *E. coli* (Engerbrecht et al. 1983).

The *luxA* and *luxB* genes encode subunits of the heterodimeric luciferase enzyme. Luciferase catalyses the oxidation of an aldehyde and reduced flavin mononucleotide, producing a long-chain fatty acid, water and flavin mononucleotide. Emission of blue–green light, with a maximum intensity at 490 nm, accompanying the oxidation reaction has led to this reaction which is known as **bioluminescence**.

Different luminescent bacteria may show differences in the luminescence spectrum and the colour of the emitted light due to sensitizer proteins that causes shift in wave length (Meighen, 1992). The initial stage of bioluminescence induction involves an interaction between OOHL, often equated with a pheromone, and the transcriptional regulator protein, *luxR. V. fischeri* cells express *luxI* at a basal level, when present in low population densities and therefore the concentration of OOHL in the medium remains low whereas with the increase in the population density within the confines of a light organ, the concentration of OOHL in the environment also increases. When the critical concentration is achieved, OOHL diffuses back into the cell and binds to *luxR.* Once the auto-inducer is bound to the N-terminal regulatory domain, multimer formation by *luxR* is enhanced and the C-terminal domain activates transcription from both the *luxR* functions probably by the OOHL mediated induction of a conformational change (Finney et al. 2002).

Expression of *luxR* is regulated by two regulatory proteins — *LuxR* and CAP regulatory proteins. Induction of transcription from *luxICDABEG* operon increases the cellular levels of mRNA transcripts required both for bioluminescence and OOHL synthesis, i.e. auto-induction. As the concentration of OOHL molecules increases, more of it diffuses back into the cell and is able to activate more *luxR* within the *V. fischeri* population. Thus, auto-induction ensures that bioluminescence and signaling molecule production continues.

However, in *V. fischeri* the intercellular communication does not lead to a radical alteration in the shape or behavior of the cells but chemical signaling in myxobacteria causes astonishing changes in structure and activity (Losick and Kaiser, 1997).

Myxobacterial Developmental Cycle

Myxococcus xanthus exists as a self-organized, predatory, saprotrophic, single-species biofilm called a swarm. *Myxococcus xanthus*, found almost ubiquitously in soil, are thin, rod, shaped, Gram-negative cells that exhibit self-organizing behavior as a response to environmental cues. The swarm, which has been compared to a "wolf-pack," modifies its environment through synergy. This behavior facilitates predatory feeding, as the concentration of extracellular digestive enzymes secreted by the bacteria increases. *M. xanthus* is a model organism for studying development in which starving bacteria self-organize to form fruiting bodies, i.e. dome-shaped structures of approximately 1,00,000 cells. These swarms differentiate into metabolically quiescent and environmentally resistant **myxospores** over the course of several days. During this process of self-organiziation, dense ridges of cells move in traveling waves (ripples) that grow and shrink over several hours.

A swarm of *M. xanthus* is a distributed system; a population of identical automata whose distribution is transparent so that the swarm appears to be one machine rather than thousands of small machines. It contains millions of cells that act as a collective, exhibiting coordinated movement through a series of signals to create dynamic patterns in response to environmental cues. One of these behaviors, i.e. development, is controlled through a cascade or series of transcriptional regulators (TR) that control downstream gene expression. It has been proposed that all emergent or self-organizing behaviors in *M. xanthus* are under this type of control.

Nutrient limitation in the presence of a solid surface and at a high cell density triggers the first steps in the developmental cycle of *M. xanthus*. The initiation and progression of aggregation involves both intracellular signals in individual cells and intercellular signals. The intracellular signals are believed to be mediated by *rel A*-dependent (p) ppGpp accumulation, since *M. xanthus* relies primarily on an amino acid-based diet, and depletion of one or more amino acids will trigger a stringent response.

Two additional factors are proposed to play a role in determining entry into the developmental cycle: the products of the *soc E* and *csg A* genes. The *soc E* gene product is unknown and does not exhibit homology to any other proteins in the databases. The *soc E* gene is highly expressed in vegetative cells and becomes depleted in non-growing starved cells as a result of inhibition by ppGpp or stringent response. It is the depletion of the *soc E* product that is believed to be important in Soc E's role in regulating the induction of the developmental cycle. Thus, it is the induction of the stringent response and the balance between *soc E* and *csgA* that appears to be important in the decision to enter into development.

Five intercellular signals A, B, C, D and E have been identified as mediators of the aggregation and fruiting body formation. The earliest acting signal involved in fruiting body and myxospore formation is the **A-signal** appears to be a mixture of both amino acids and peptides that are generated by proteases secreted by the myxobacteria. Generation of the A-signal involves at least three genes—*asgA* (*asg*, meaning A-signal gene), *asgB*, and *asgC*. Other signals include: (1) the **B-signal** which acts early in the development, has not been yet identified. It is dependent on the *bsgA* gene product; (2) the **C-signal** which is a 17 Kda and a 25 Kda protein encoded by the *csgA* gene. It is the most extensively characterized signal, essential for directed motility during aggregation and fruiting body formation also for differentiation into myxospores. Both proteins are cell surface associated. It is positively regulated by *(p) ppGpp* and positively regulates *relA*; (3) the **D-signal**, the least understood of the extracellular signals, which is believed to be a mixture of fatty acids and is dependent on the *dsgA* gene; and (4) the **E-signal**, which appears to be long branched-chain fatty acids and requires the *esgA* and *esgB* gene products. Its product is homologue of the *E. coli* initiation factor (IF)-3. They are believed to play a role in generating E-signals from fatty acids in the environment.

Response to, and for some the production of these extracellular signals (A-, B-, C-, D-and E-signals) requires high cell densities. High cell densities are essential for the effective exchange and response to cell signals as well as necessary direct cell-to-cell interactions (Moat et al. 2002).

Cell surface appendages are called **fibrils**. Fibrils are filamentous structures up to 50 μm long and are composed of polysaccharides and closely associated **integral fibril proteins (IFPs)**. Fibrils are important for cell-to-cell cohesion and the characteristic social behaviour associated with the developmental cycle.

S-motility is not a random process. In both vegetative swarming and developmental aggregation, cells respond chemotactically, moving toward attractants (nutrients) and away from repellents. One such attractant is phosphatidylethanolamine (PE), both dilauroyl and dioleoyl PE. At least two signal transduction systems play a role in developmental aggregation—the **Frz** and **Dif systems**. The Dif system functions early in the aggregation process, since *dif* (defect in fruiting) mutants fail to aggregate beyond the early stages of fruiting body formation. The *Frz* system functions in both vegetative swarming activity and at later stages in fruiting body formation (Moat et al. 2002).

Fruiting Body Formation

Fruiting body formation is initiated by the presence of three conditions—nutrient limitation, solid surface, and high cell density. These conditions lead to accumulation of the intracellular signal *(p) ppGpp*, which in turn regulates the transcription of genes necessary for the production of the first developmental signal—A-signal. Based on evidence to date, the generation of these two signals is required for the initiation of development and fruiting body formation. Within a few hours following the onset of starvation, cells begin to aggregate, forming aggregation centers.

However, all signaling between bacteria and higher organisms does not work to the benefit of both. Disease causing species transmit chemical signals that instruct the cells of a host to alter their behaviour. But in the case of pathogens, the signals elicit responses that are detrimental to the host, disabling its defenses and enabling the pathogens to gain a foothold (Losick and Kaiser, 1997).

Many diverse microorganisms, both Gram-negative and Gram-positive, use quorum-sensing systems to regulate phenotypes ranging from mating to virulence against the host, antibiotics and production of other metabolites (Dunny and Winans, 1999).

Virulence in some Gram-negative Bacteria

Virulence of many Gram-negative members is regulated by quorum-sensing (Kievit and Iglweski, 2000). A number of studies have been reported on *Pseudomonas aeruginosa*, an opportunistic human pathogen that produces and secretes multiple extracellular virulence factors that cause extensive host tissue damage. Production of virulence factors is under the hierarchial control of two pairs of *luxI/luxR* homologues, *lasI/lasR* (Pesci et al. 1997) and *RhlI/RhlR* (Brint et al. 1995). Both *lasI* and *RhlI* are autoinducer synthases that catalyse the formation of HSLs, N-(3-oxododecanoyl)-homoserine lactone (OdDHL) and N-(butanoyl)-homoserine lactone (BHL), respectively (Pearson et al. 1995). A third autoinducer has been recently demonstrated to be involved in quorum-sensing in *P. aeruginosa*. The signal, 2-heptyl-3-hydroxy-4-quinolone or PQS (*Pseudomonas* quinolone signal) is unique because it does not fall under the category of homoserine lactones (Pesci et al. 1999).

Burkholderia cepacia, which is an emerging pathogen in cystic fibrosis patients usually as a coinfecting agent with *P. aeruginosa*. *B. cepacia* possesses both *luxR* and *luxI* homologues called *CepR* and *CepI*, respectively. The same conditions that lead to the accumulation of *P. aeruginosa* AHLs result in a 1000-fold less amount of *B. cepacia* AHL. It has been reported that *P. aeruginosa*. AHLs can increase the pathogenicity of *B. cepacia.*

Both, *E. coli* and *Salmonella enterica* serovar. *typhimurium*, possess a *luxR* homologue encoded by the *SdiA* gene. Virulence genes regulated by *Sdi A* in enteropathogenic *E. coli* (EHEC) include the genes encoding *EspD* and intimin, both of which are negatively regulated by *SdiA*. The SdiA-AI complex was determined to positively regulate four genes on the *S. typhimurium* virulence plasmid that appear to compose an operon (Michael et al. 2001).

The plant pathogen *Erwinia carotovora* also employs quorum sensing to control virulence factors during their pathogenesis in plants. The regulation of the exoenzymes is cell density dependent and controlled by the *luxR/luxI* homologues, *ExpR* and *ExpI*. Additionally *E. carotovora* possesses a second quorum-sensing system involved in the production of the antibiotic *carbapenem*. This second quorum-sensing system involves the *CarR* and *CarI*, *luxR/luxI* homologues.

Agrobacterium tumefaciens uses quorum-sensing to mediate conjugal transfer of its Ti plasmid. The Ti plasmid is also a conjugative plasmid possessing *tra* genes capable of mediating its transfer via conjugation between bacterial cells. *TraR* protein, a *luxR* homologue and an autoinducer synthase *TraI* positively control conjugal transfer of the Ti plasmid (Pierson et al. 1999).

Quorum-sensing in some Gram-positive Bacteria

The quorum-sensing systems of Gram-positive bacteria are fundamentally different from those of Gram-negative bacteria. They do not produce AHL and use sensor–kinase/regulator two-component signal transduction systems. They produce peptide signals that interact with sensor kinase, which then phosphorylates the cognate regulator protein (Dunny et al. 1997).

Quorum-sensing is used to regulate the development of bacterial competence in *Bacillus subtilis* and *Streptococcus pneumoniae*, conjugation in *Streptococcus faecalis*, and virulence in *Staphylococcus aureus*. *S. aureus* produces an impressive collection of virulence factors expressed at stages during infection. Initially, bacterium synthesizes a number of surface-associated factors involved in adherence to host tissues and host defense evasion. The successive regulation of virulence factors is under the control of two regulatory loci: *agr* (accessory gene regulator) and *sar* (staphylococcal accessory gene regulator). The *agr* locus contains two divergently transcribed operons encoding two polysistronic mRNAs referred to as RNAII and RNAIII. The *agr* BDCA operon (RNAII) encodes *agrC*, a signal transducer protein, and *agrA*, a response regulator. *agrB* and *agrD* are involved in producing the quorum-sensing signal molecule. RNAIII encodes the δ-hemolysin and also functions as a regulatory RNA molecule. During quorum-sensing, *agrC* binds to the peptide signal molecule, phosphorylates itself (autophosphorylation), and then phosphorylates *agrA*. Phospho-*agrA* (*agrA-P*) then induces RNAIII expression, which goes on to stimulate the expression of numerous secreted products and to downregulate specific surface protein expression as well as increase the expression of *agrBDCA*.

CONCLUSION

In this chapter, an overview of why and how bacteria communicate has been discussed with the help of some of the best studied and most intriguing examples of cell signaling. Bacteria communicate with the help of chemical signal molecule (autoinducers). The quorum-sensing enables bacteria to count the members in the vicinal community and, in response to changes in population density and alter the gene expression. No single system operates independently in the cell, there are several layers of control that monitor and modulate the expression of any given gene. It is very important to explore the methods which can enhance or decrease the signaling cascade as it can be used for finding the solutions to the problems like plant and animal diseases, regulation of useful as well as toxic fermentation products, to track multiple resistance for drugs in clinical pathogens, biofilm formation in surgical equipments and other aspects of pathogenicity.

In the environment, the conversations that bacteria hold with their neighbours await further and exciting discoveries of great value to humankind.

REFERENCES

1. Brint JM, Ohman DE. Synthesis of multiple exoproducts in *Pseudonomas aeruginosa* is under the control of RlR-RhlI, another set of regulators in strain PAO-I with homology to the autoinducer-responsive LuxR-LuxI family. *J Bacteriol.*, 1995, 177, 7155–7163.

2. D. De Kievit TR, Iglweski BH. Bacterial quorum-sensing in pathogenic relationships. *Infect. Immun.*, 2000, 68, 4839–4849.

3. Dunny GM, Leonard BAB 1997. Cell-cell communication in gram positive bacteria. *Annu. Rev. Microbiol.*, 51:527–64.

4. Dunny, G. M. and Winans, S. C., *Cell-Cell Signalling in Bacteria* (eds Dunny, G. M. and Winans, S. C.), ASM Press, Washington, 1999, pp. 1–5.

5. Engebrecht, J., Nealson, K. L. and Silverman, M. Bacterial bioluminescence: isolation and genetic analysis of the functions from *Vibriio fischeri. Cell*, 1983, 32, 773–781.

6. Engerbrecht, J. and Silverman, M. Nucleotide sequence of the regulatory locus controlling expression of bacterial genes for bioluminescence. *Nucletic Acids Res.* 1987, 15, 10455–10467.

7. Fuqua, C. and Eberhard ,A. Cell-Cell Signaling in Bacteria, ASM Press, Washington, 1999, pp.211–230.

8. Hastings, J. W and Greenberg, E. P., Quorum sensing: the explanation of a curious phenomenon reveals a common characteristic of bacteria. *J. Bacteriol.*, 1999, 181, 2667–2668.

9. Henderson B., Wilson M., McNab R., Lax A.J. Cellular Microbiology: Bacterial-Host Interactions in Health and Disease. Cellular Microbiology, 2001, 112–117.

10. Losick, R.,Kaiser, D., Why and How bacteria Communicate, Scientific American, 1997, 52–57.

11. Meighen, E. A., *Encyclopedia of Microbiology* (ed. Leaderberg, J.), Academic Press, 1992, pp. 309–319.

12. Melissa, B., Miller. Bonnie L. B, Quorum Sensing in Bacteria. Annual Review of Microbiology. 2001, 55, 165–199.

13. Michael. B, J. N. Smith, S. Swift, F. Heffron and B. M. Ahmer. SdiA of *Salmonella enteric*a in a LuxR homolog that detects mixed microbial communities. *J. Bacteriol.*, 2001, 183:5733–42.

14. Moat A.G., Foster J.W., Spector M.P. Microbial Physiology, 2002, 4:234–236.

15. Pearson, J P , Passador, L., Iglewski, N .H. and Greenburg, E P , A second N-acyllhomoserine lactone signal product produced by *Pseudonomas aeruginosa. Proc. Natl. Acad. Sci. USA, 1995*, 95, 1490–1494.

16. Perbal ,B.,Cell communication and signaling 2003, 1:3 doi:10.1186/1478-11 x-1-3.

17. Pesci, EC , Pearson, J P Seed, P C and Iglewski, B H , Regulation of *las* and *rhl* quorum sensing in *Pseudonomas aeruginosa, J Bacterial.*, 1997, 179,3127–3132.

18. Pesci, EC, Milbank, J B J, Pearson, J P, Mcknoght, S, Kende A S, Greenberg, E P and Iglewski, B H., Quinolone signaling in cell-to-cell communication system of *Pseudonomas aeruginosa, Proc. Natl. Acad. Sci. USA, 1999*, 96, 11229–11234.

19. Pesci,EC.,Pearson, J.P.,Seed, P.C. and Iglewski,B.H., Regulation of las and rhl quorumsensing in pseudomonas aaeruginosa. J. Bacteriol., 1997, 179, 3127–3132.

20. Pierson, L.Sm, III, D.W. Wood, and S Beck von Bonman. Quorum- sensing in plant-associated bacteria. In G.M. Dunny and S C Winans (eds.), *Cell-Cell Signaling in Bacteria.* American Society for Microbiology Press, Washington, DC, 1999, pp. 101–16.

21. Whitehead, NA., Barnard, A. M. L., Slater, H., Simpson, N. J. L. and Salmond, G. P. C., Quorum-sensing in Gram-negative bacteria. *FEMS Microbiol. Rev.* 2001, 25, 365–404.

4

Bacteriocins from Lactic Acid Bacteria: Classification, Production, Purification and Inventory Potential Applications

Tejpal Dhewa • Shailja Pant • Shailesh K Joshi

INTRODUCTION

The classification of lactic acid bacteria (LAB) was initiated in 1919 by Orla-Jensen and was until recently primary based on morphological, metabolic and physiological criteria. LAB comprise a diverse group of Gram-positive, non-spore forming, non-motile rod-and coccus-shaped catalase-lacking organisms. They are chemo-organotrophic and only grow in complex media. Fermentable carbohydrates and higher alcohols are used as the energy source to form chiefly lactic acid. LAB degrade hexoses to lactate (homofermentative) or lactate and additional products such as acetate, ethanol, CO_2, formate or succinate (heterofermentative). They are widely distributed in different ecosystems and are commonly found in foods (dairy products, fermented meats and vegetables, sourdough, silage, beverages), sewage, on plants but also in the genital, intestinal and respiratory tracts of man and animals. Current methodologies used for classification of LAB mainly rely on 16S ribosomal ribonucleic acid (rRNA) analysis and sequencing. Based on these techniques, Gram-positive bacteria are divided into two groups depending on their G + C content. The Actinomycetes have a G + C content above 50 mol% and contain genera such as *Atopobium*, *Bifidobacterium*, *Corynebacterium* and *Propionibacterium*. In contrast, the Clostridium branch has a G + C content below 50 mol% and include the typical LAB genera *Carnobacterium*, *Lactobacillus*, *Lactococcus*, *Leuconostoc*, *Pediococcus* and *Streptococcus*. Lactic acid bacteria have a long history of application in fermented foods because of their beneficial influence on nutritional, organoleptic, and shelf-life characteristics (Wood and Holzapfel, 1995). They cause rapid acidification of the raw material through the production of organic acids, mainly lactic acid. In addition, their production of acetic acid, ethanol, aroma compounds, bacteriocins, exoploysaccharides, and several enzymes is of importance. Whereas a food fermentation process with LAB is traditionally based on spontaneous fermentation or backs lopping, industrial food fermentation is nowadays performed by the deliberate addition of LAB as starter cultures to the food matrix. This has been a breakthrough in the processing of fermented foods, resulting in a high degree of control over the fermentation process and standardization of the end products. Recently, the use of functional starter cultures, a novel generation of starter cultures that offers functionalities beyond acidification, is being explored (Leroy and De Vuyst, 2004; Leroy et al. 2006; De Vuyst et al. 2004). For instance, LAB are capable of inhibiting various microorganisms in a food environment and display crucial antimicrobial properties with respect to food preservation and safety. In addition, it has been shown that some strains of LAB possess interesting health-promoting properties; one of the characteristics of these probiotics is the potential to combat gastrointestinal pathogenic bacteria such as *Helicobacter pylori*, *Escherichia coli*, and *Salmonella* (Fig. 4.1).

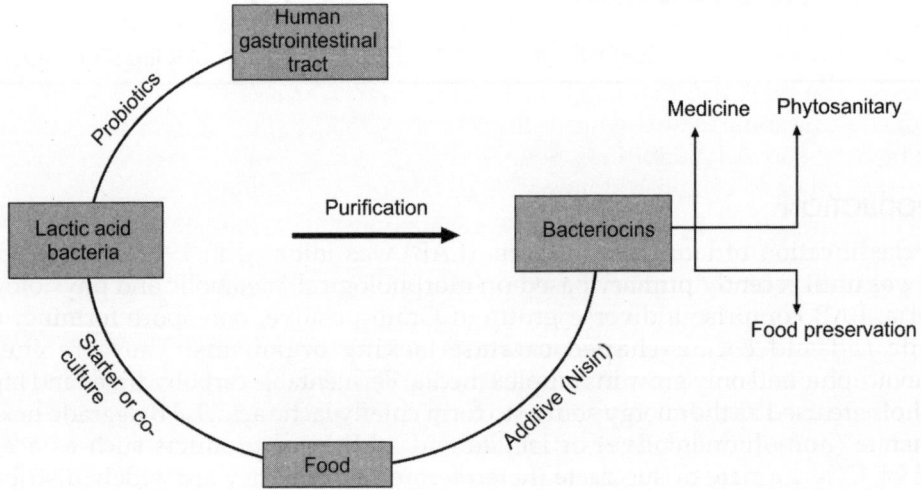

Fig. 4.1: Overview of the application potential of bacteriocin production by LAB

Antimicrobial Property of Lactic Acid Bacteria

LAB display a wide range of antagonistic activities, i. e. the production of lactic acid, acetic acid, bioactive molecules such as ethanol, formic acid, fatty acids, hydrogen peroxide, diacetyl, reuterin, and reutericyclin. Many strains also produce bacteriocins and bacteriocin-like molecules that display antibacterial activity (De Vuyst and Vandamme, 1994). Bacteriocins are proteinaceous toxins produced by bacteria to inhibit the growth of similar or closely related bacterial strain (s). They are typically considered to be narrow spectrum antibiotics, though this has been debated (Farkas-Himsley, 1980). Besides the production of bacteriocins, some LAB are able to synthesize other antimicrobial peptides that may also contribute to food preservation and safety. For instance, strains of *Lactobacillus plantarum*, isolated from sourdough and grass silage, display antifungal activity, due to the production of organic acids, other low-molecular-mass metabolites, and/or cyclic dipeptides (Lavermicocca et al. 2000; Strøm et al. 2002; Schnürer and Magnusson, 2005). It is not unlikely that additional, new antimicrobial peptides are to be discovered (Makras et al. 2006). Although still in its infancy, there is good reason to believe that genomics will soon become an essential tool for exploring the antimicrobial potency of LAB (Nes and Johnsborg, 2004). Interestingly, bacteriocin screening programs have yielded, during the last decades, a large arsenal of bacteriocins with different properties, target species, and producer organisms (Cotter et al. 2006).

Lactic Acid Bacteria as Probiotics

Lactic acid bacteria were referred to as probiotics in scientific literature. The most recent and accurate description of probiotics was undertaken by Fuller (1989) who redefined it as "a live microbial feed supplement beneficial to the host (man or animal) by improving the microbial balance within its body". Another definition is "probiotics as viable microbial food supplements which beneficially influence the health of the host". The gastrointestinal tract contains food in different stages of digestion, digestive ferments, liquids and solid waste. Within the gut are also wide ranges of microbes that may be either harmful or beneficial. The beneficial ones assist in the breakdown of food while they also manufacture vitamins essential to the body, breaking down and destroying some toxic chemicals that may have been ingested with the food. Under both healthy and sick conditions, several different types of bacteria compete or fight with each other to establish dominance in the warm and moist environment of the alimentary canal that serves as an ecosystem for their survival and propagation. The average human large intestine harbors over 400 different species of bacteria with a total population far outnumbering even the number of human cells in the body. Under ideal conditions of health and diet, the different strains of bacteria on microflora compete and check the excessive number of any one strain. Healthy condition can be achieved, if a balance is maintained between the "good" and "bad" bacteria in the ratio of 85% to 15%. Oral supplement of diet with viable *Lactobacillus acidophilus* of human origin, which is bile resistant, led to a significant decline of three different fecal bacterial enzymes. This decrease in the fecal bacterial enzyme activity observed in both humans and rats included beta glucuronidase, azoreductase and nitroreductase. All these enzymes catalyse the conversion of procarcinogens to proximal carcinogens in the large bowel leading to colon cancer. Lactic acid bacteria including *Lactobacillus, Leuconostoc, Lactococcus, Pediococcus* and *Bifidobacterium* are found throughout the gastrointestinal tract. The predominant population of lactic acid bacteria in the upper gastrointestinal tract is the *Lactobacillus* species which may colonize the mucosal surface of the duodenum as well as the stomach. *Lactobacillus* and *Bifidobacterium* sp. are prominent members of the commensal intestinal flora and are the commonly studied probiotics bacteria. They cause reduced lactose intolerance alleviation of some diarrhoeas, lowered blood cholesterol, increased immune response and prevention of cancer. The selection criteria for probiotic LAB include: human origin, safety, viability/ activity in delivery vehicles, resistance to acid and bile, adherence to gut epithelial tissue, ability to colonise the gastrointestinal tract, production of antimicrobial substances, ability to stimulate a host immune response and the ability to influence metabolic activities such as vitamin production, cholesterol assimilation and lactose activity (Dhewa et al. 2010; Dhewa and Goyal, 2009; Dhewa et al. 2009 a; Dhewa et al.,

2009b; Puniya et al. 2008). Fuller (1989) listed the following organisms as species used in probiotic preparation: *Lactobacillus acidophilus, Lactobacillus casei, Lactobacillus casei* subsp. *rhamnosus, Lactobacillus fermentum, Lactobacillus reuteri, Lactococcus lactis subsp. lactis, Lactococcus lactis subsp. cremoris, Lactobacillus bulgaricus, Lactobacillus plantarum, Streptococcus thermophilus, Enterococcus faecium, Enterococcus faecalis, Bifidobacterium bifidum, Bifidobacterium infantis, Bifidobacterium adolescentis, Bifidobacterium longum, Bifidobacterium breve.*

BACTERIOCINS: CLASSIFICATION

Bacteriocins were first discovered by A. Gratia in 1925 (Gratia, 1925; Gratia, 2000), the term "colicine" was coined by Gratia and Fredericq (1946); "bacteriocine" was used by Jacob et al. (1953) as a general term for highly specific antibacterial proteins. The term colicin now implies a bacteriocidal protein produced by varieties of *E. coli* and closely related Enterobacteriaceae (Konisky, 1982). Bacteriocins (as colicins) were originally defined as bactericidal proteins characterized by lethal biosynthesis, a very narrow range of activity, and adsorption to specific cell envelope receptors (Jacob et al. 1953). Later, the recognized association of bacteriocin biosynthesis with plasmids was added to the description. The definition has since been modified to incorporate the properties of bacteriocins produced by Gram-positive bacteria (Tagg et al. 1976). Bacteriocins from Gram-positive bacteria commonly do not possess a specific receptor for adsorption although exceptions exist (Gravesen et al. 2002), are most frequently of lower molecular weight than colicins, have a broader range of target bacteria with different modes of release and cell transport, and possess leader sequences cleaved during maturation (Jack et al. 1995; James et al. 1991; Riley, 1998). Nowadays, bacteriocidal peptides or proteins produced by bacteria are typically referred to as bacteriocins. Typically, to demonstrate the proteinaceous nature of a newly characterized bacteriocin, sensitivity to proteolytic enzymes such as trypsin, chymotrypsin, and pepsin is an expected demonstration. Evaluation for use as a food additive requires estimation of its heat resistance given the widespread use of thermal processing in food production. Over the years, several publications have reviewed colicins, bacteriocins, bacteriocins from LAB, and applications of specific bacteriocins. Examples include Reeves (1972), Franklin and Snow (1975), Hardy (1975), Tagg et al. (1976), Konisky (1982), Klaenhammer (1988, 1993), Jack et al. (1995), de Vos et al. (1995), Sahl et al. (1995), Venema et al., (1995), Abee et al. (1995), and Cleveland et al. (2001). Most of the bacteriocins from LAB are cationic, hydrophobic, or amphiphilic molecules composed of 20 to 60 amino acid residues. These bacteriocins are commonly classified into 3 groups that also include bacteriocins from other Gram-positive bacteria (Klaenhammer, 1993, Nes et al. 1996). Examples of bacteriocins from these 3 classes are summarized in Table 4.1.

1. Class I contained antibiotics (from lanthionine-containing antibiotic) are small (<5 kDa) peptides containing the unusual amino acids lanthionine (Lan), methyllanthionine (MeLan), dehydroalanine, and dehydrobutyrine. It is further subdivided into type A and type B lantibiotics according to chemical structures (Fig. 4.2) and antimicrobial activities (Moll et al. 1999; van Kraaij et al. 1999; Guder et al., 2000).
   (i) Type A: Lantibiotics are elongated peptides with a net positive charge that exert their activity through the formation of pores in bacterial membranes, and (ii) Type B:

Lantibiotics are smaller globular peptides and have a negative or no net charge; antimicrobial activity is related to the inhibition of specific enzymes.

Table 4.1: Examples of bacteriocins (Chen and Hoover, 2003)

Bacteriocins	Producer	References
Class I-type A lantibiotics		
Nisin	*Lactococcus lactis*	Hurst, 1981
Lactocin S	*Lactobacillus sake*	Mortvedt et al. 1991
Epidermin	*Staphylococcus*	Allgaier et al. 1986
Gallidermin	*epidermidis*	Kellner et al. 1988
Lacticin 481	*Staphylococcus*	Piard et al. 1992
	gallinarum	
	L. lactis	
Class I-type B lantibiotics		
Mersacidin	*Bacillus subtilis*	Altena et al. 2000
Cinnamycin	*Streptomyces*	Sahl and Bierbaum, 1998
Ancovenin	*cinnamoneus*	Sahl and Bierbaum, 1998
Duramycin	*Streptomyces* sp.	Sahl and Bierbaum, 1998
Actagardin	*S. cinnamoneus*	Sahl and Bierbaum, 1998
	Actinoplanes sp.	
Class IIa		
pediocin PA-1/AcH	*Pediococcus acidilactici*	Henderson et al. 1992; Motlagh et al. 1992
Sakacin A	*L. sake*	Holck et al. 1992
Sakacin P	*L. sake*	Tichaczek et al. 1992
Leucocin A-UAL 187	*Leuconostoc gelidum*	Hastings et al. 1991
Mesentericin Y 105	*Leuconostoc*	Hechard et al. 1992
Enterocin A	*mesenteroides*	Aymerich et al. 1996
Divercin V 41	*Enterococcus faecium*	Metivier et al. 1998
Lactococcin MMFII	*Carnobacterium divergens*	Ferchichi et al. 2001
	L. lactis	
Class IIb		
Lactococcin G	*L. lactis*	Nissen-Meyer et al. 1992
Lactococcin M	*L. lactis*	van Belkum et al. 1991
Lactacin F	*Lactobacillus johnsonii*	Allison et al. 1994
Plantaricin A	*Lactobacillus plantarum*	Nissen-Meyer et al. 1993
Plantaricin S	*L. plantarum*	imenez-Diaz et al. 1995
Plantaricin EF	*L. plantarum*	J Anderssen et al. 1998
Plantaricin JK	*L. plantarum*	Anderssen et al. 1998
Class IIc		
Acidocin B	*Lactobacillus acidophilus*	Leer et al. 1995
Carnobacteriocin A	*Carnobacterium piscicola*	Worobo et al. 1994
Divergicin A	*C. divergens*	Worobo et al. 1995
Enterocin P	*E. faecium*	Cintas et al. 1998
Enterocin B	*E. faecium*	Nes and Holo, 2000
Class III		
Helveticin J	*Lactobacillus helveticus*	Joerger and Klaenhammer, 1986
Helveticin V-1829	*L. helveticus*	Vaughan et al. 1992

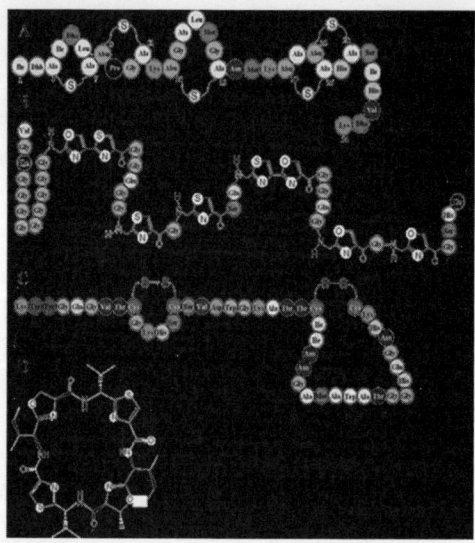

Fig. 4.2: Covalent structure of some representative peptide-bacteriocins. A: nisin, B: microcin B17, C: pediocin PA-1, D: patellamide A (desriac et al. 2010).

2. Class II includes small (<10 kDa), heat-stable, non-lanthionine-containing peptides. The largest group of bacteriocins in this classification system, these peptides are divided into 3 subgroups: (i) Class IIa: includes pediocin-like peptides having an N-terminal consensus sequence-Tyr-Gly-Asn-Gly-Val-Xaa-Cys. This subgroup has attracted much of the attention due to their anti-Listeria activity (Ennahar et al., 2000). (ii) Class IIb: contains bacteriocins requiring 2 different peptides for activity, and (iii) Class IIc: includes the remaining peptides of the class, including sec-dependent secreted bacteriocins.
3. Class III bacteriocins are not as well characterized. It houses large (>30 kDa) heat-labile proteins that are of lesser interest to food scientists.

A 4th class consisting of complex bacteriocins that require carbohydrate or lipid moieties for activity has also been suggested by Klaenhammer (1993); however, bacteriocins in this class have not been characterized adequately at the biochemical level to the extent that the definition of this class requires additional descriptive information (Jimenez-Diaz et al. 1995; McAuliffe et al. 2001).

Databases

Two databases of bacteriocins are available: BAGEL (de Jong et al. 2006) and BACTIBASE (Hammami et al. 2007; Hammami et al. 2010).

Bacteriocin Specificity

Bacteriocins are unique antimicrobial peptides. Indeed, the producing strain has to protect itself from its own peptides, so bacteriocin-producing bacteria have to develop some sort of immunity strategy. In addition to a structural gene, post-translational gene and export machinery, the gene cluster organization of bacteriocin encodes as well for an immunity protein. The latter ensures bacteriocin protection in various ways, depending on the bacteriocin mechanism of action. Immunity to pore forming colicins is mediated by an 11 to 18 kDa small membrane protein. A direct and specific interaction within the inner membrane between the immunity protein and the C-terminal part of colicin achieves cell protection. Transmembrane helices have been shown to be the main motifs recognized by immunity proteins. Colicins targeting intracellular enzymes such as nuclease are inactivated by direct binding of the immunity protein (about 10 kDa) to the active domain of colicin leading to a 71 kDa heterodimer (Desriac et al. 2010).

BACTERIOCINS: PRODUCTION AND PURIFICATIONS

Though bacteriocins can be produced in the food matrix during food fermentation, bacteriocins by LAB can be produced in much higher amounts during in vitro fermentations under optimal physical and chemical conditions (Leroy and De Vuyst, 2005). The higher in vitro production is due to the absence of limiting factors, such as strong diffusion limitations, inactivation by proteases, and the adsorption to food particles (Leroy and De Vuyst, 2000). However, even during controlled fermentor experiments, considerable differences in activity yields are obtained, and an influence of the environmental process conditions on the obtained bacteriocin activity can be seen. For instance, a decrease of pH results in a decreased adsorption of the bacteriocin molecules to the producer cells, and hence in an increased bioavailability (Yang et al. 1992). In addition, temperature and pH (Lejeune et al., 1998; Leroy and De Vuyst, 1999; Van den Berghe et al. 2006) as well as nutrient availability (Callewaert and De Vuyst, 2000) seem to play a crucial role in bacteriocin production, whereas the presence of elevated amounts of sodium chloride usually decreases production levels. In general, the cultivation conditions directly affect bacteriocin production as such (specific bacteriocin production in particular) and, indirectly, through biomass production. This is to be explained by the fact that bacteriocin production is a growth-dependent physiological trait and hence follows primary metabolite kinetics (De Vuystn et al. 1996; Lejeune et al. 1998).

Three major methods for the purification of bacteriocins by LAB to homogeneity can be distinguished. First, purification can be done by a conventional method that is based on a rather laborious series of subsequent steps of ammonium sulfate precipitation, ion exchange, hydrophobic interaction, gel filtration, and reversed-phase high-pressure liquid chromatography (Mørtvedt et al., 1991; Tichaczek et al., 1992; Parente and Ricciardi, 1999). Second, a simple three-step protocol has been developed (Callewaert et al. 1999), including: (i) ammonium sulfate precipitation, (ii) chloroform/methanol extraction/precipitation, and (iii) reversed-phase high-pressure liquid chromatography, the sole chromatographic step involved. Third, bacteriocins can be isolated through a unique unit operation, i.e. expanded bed adsorption, using a hydrophobic interaction gel, after maximizing the bioavailable bacteriocin titer through pH adjustment of the crude fermentation medium (Callewaert and De Vuyst, 1999; Foulquié Moreno et al., 2001). Following the latter two methods, which are more rapid than the first conventional method and yet successful, several bacteriocins with interesting industrial potential have been purified, such as the class II bacteriocins amylovorin L (produced by *Lactobacillus amylovorus* DCE 471) and several enterocins (produced by the *Enterococcus faecium* RZS C5, RZS C13, and FAIR-E 406 strains), and the lantibiotic macedocin (produced by *Streptococcus macedonicus* ACA-DC 198)

(Callewaert and De Vuyst,1999; Foulquié Moreno et al. 2002; Foulquié Moreno et al. 2003; Georgalaki et al. 2002; De Vuyst and Leroy, 2007).

BACTERIOCINS: POTENTIAL APPLICATIONS

Bacteriocins from LAB have demonstrated their remarkable potential as food conservatives (Rihakova et al. 2009) or as therapeutics for veterinary or medical uses (Tagg et al. 2003) or as phytosanitary for plant protection (Holtsmark et al. 2008). Bacteriocins are of interest in medicine because they are made by non-pathogenic bacteria that normally colonize the human body:

- Bacteriocins have also been suggested as a cancer treatment (Farkas-Himsley and Yu 1985; Baumal et al., 1982; Saito et.al. 1979; Cruz-Chamorro et al. 2006; Sand et al. 2007; Farkas-Himsley et al. 1995; Musclow et al. 1987). Partly this is due to questions about their mechanism of action and the presumption that antibacterial agents have no obvious connection to killing mammalian tumor cells.
- In the long quest for medical applications, bacteriocins have also been tested as AIDS drugs (Farkas-Himsley et al. 1991).

Bacteriocins can be used as food additives. For instance, nisin is commercially made in a partially purified form and a marketed preparation with the pediocin PA-1 (AcH) producer is available. Schillinger et al. (1996) described three common approaches used in the application of bacteriocins for biopreservation of foods:

  i. Inoculation of food with LAB that produce bacteriocin in the products.

  ii. Addition of purified or semi-purified bacteriocins as food preservatives, i.e. biopreservation of dairy products, meat, seafood and packaging film.

  iii. Use of a product previously fermented with a bacteriocin producing strain as an ingredient in food processing.

As an alternative to the addition of bacteriocins to foods, bacteriocins may be produced directly in the food as a result of starter culture or co-culture activity. Several studies have indeed indicated that LAB starter cultures or co-cultures are able to produce their bacteriocins in food matrices, and consequently display inhibitory activity towards sensitive food spoilage or pathogenic bacteria. The latter trait has mainly been documented for fermented sausage, fermented vegetables and olives, and dairy products. For instance; bacteriocin extraction has been demonstrated in the case of Cheddar cheese and fermented sausage and sourdough. Application of bacteriocin-producing starter cultures in sourdough (to increase competitiveness and hence establish a desired microbial population), in fermented sausage (anti-listerial effect to meet the zero-tolerance policy in ready-to-eat foods), and in cheese (anti-listerial and anti-clostridial effects), have been studied during in vitro laboratory fermentations as well as on pilot-scale level (Leroy and De Vuyst, 2005; Foulquié Moreno et al. 2003; Anastasiou et al. 2006).

This is remarkable considering the obvious potential that bacteriocins or bacteriocin-producing strains have for plant disease control and considering the fact that both genome analyses and experimental studies (Hu and Young, 1998) indicate that bacteriocins are also abundantly present in plant pathogens (Holtsmark et al., 2008). Some examples are:

- *Rhizobium leguminosarum* produces such an RTX-type toxin of about 100 kDa, provides a competitive advantage (in terms of nodule occupancy) in the competition with some (not all) closely related strains (Oresnik et al. 1999).

- *Xanthomonas perforans* produces a protein (bacteriocins) enables to exert an antagonistic effect on the tomato pathogen *Xanthomonas euvesicatoria*, both in the laboratory and in field trials (Hert et al. 2005).
- *Pectobacterium carotovorum* produces carotovoricins (bacteriocins) that kill other *Pectobacterium carotovorum* strains and that the killing spectra of these bacteriocins are determined by the structure of the tail fibers (Nguyen et al. 2001; Yamada et al. 2006). Phage-tail-like bacteriocins have also been found in *Ralstonia solanacearum* (previously *Pseudomonas solanacearum*) (Arwiyanto et al. 1993) and it has been shown that avirulent bacteriocin producers reduce the development of bacterial wilt on tobacco (Chen and Echandi, 1984).
- *Xanthomonas campestris* pv. glycines, the causative agent of bacterial pustule on soybean, produces a heterodimeric bacteriocin called glycinecin (encoded by two separate genes, glyA and glyB, 39 and a 14-kDa), which has an antagonistic activity against other pathovars of *X. campestris,* and also *X. oryzae pv. oryzae*, which causes bacterial blight of rice (Heu et al. 2001).
- Interestingly, two lectin-like bacteriocins with similar inhibitory spectra were identified in the well-known biocontrol strain *Pseudomonas fluorescens* Pf-5 (Parret et al. 2005).

Results of above studies are highly promising and emphasize the important role that bacteriocinogenic strains of LAB may play in the food industry as starter cultures, co-cultures, or bioprotective cultures, to improve food quality safety and medicine as well as phytosanitary.

CONCLUSION

This chapter gives an overview of LAB bacteriocin classifications, production, purifications and food applications. Bacteriocins produced by LAB have the potential to cover a very broad field of application, including both the food industry and the medical sector. Concerning their use in food, bacteriocin-producing starter or co-cultures have been successfully applied in pilot-scale experiments (cheese, fermented sausage, sourdough, etc.) yielding food quality and food safety advantages. With respect to medical applications, antimicrobials produced by probiotic LAB might play a role during in vivo interactions occurring in the human gastrointestinal tract, hence contributing to gut health. Further research is needed to unravel the precise role of LAB bacteriocins in this process. In recent years, LAB bacteriocins have generated interest due to their potential as a safe biopreservatives that could, at least partially, replace chemical preservatives. Although intensive studies over the last decade have greatly advanced our knowledge base about bacteriocins, further work is needed before we are able to fully understand the molecular mechanisms, structure–function relationships, and mechanisms of action of bacteriocins. Research in these areas is critical for the effective applications of bacteriocins and would help develop methods to genetically engineer bacteriocins with better activity, solubility, stability and future applications.

REFERENCES

1. Abee T, Krockel L, Hill C. 1995. Bacteriocins: modes of action and potentials in food preservation and control of food poisoning. *International Journal of Food Microbiology* 28:169–185.

2. Allgaier H, Jung G, Werner GG, et al. 1986. Epidermin: sequencing of a heterodettetracyclic 21-peptide amide antibiotic. *European Journal of Biochemistry* 160: 9–22.

3. Allison GE, Fremaux C, Klaenhammer, TR. 1994. Expansion of bacteriocin activity and host range upon complementation of 2 peptides encoded within the lactacin F operon. *Journal of Bacteriology* 176: 2235–41.

4. Altena, K., Guder, A., Cramer, C. and Bierbaum, G. 2000. Biosynthesis of the lantibiotic mersacidin: organization of a type B lantibiotic gene cluster. *Applied Environmental Microbiolology* 66:2565–71.

5. Ames, R. Lazdunski, C. and Pattus, F. 1991. *Bacteriocins, Micrococins and Lantibiotics.* New York: Springer-Verlag. pp.519.

6. Anastasiou, R. Georgalaki, M., Manolopoulou, E., Kandarakis, I., De Vuyst, L. and Tsakalidou, E. 2006. The performance of Streptococcus macedonicus ACA-DC 198 as starter culture in Kasseri cheese production. *International Dairy Journal* 17: 208–217.

7. Anderssen, E. L., Diep, D. B., Nes, I. F., Eijsink, V. G. H. and Nissen-Meijer, J. 1998. Antagonistic activity of Lactobacillus plantarum C11: 2 new 2-peptide bacteriocins, plantaricins EF and JK, and the induction factor plantaricin A. *Applied Environmental Microbiology* 6:2269–72.

8. Arwiyanto, T., Goto, M. and Takikawa, Y. 1993. Characteristics of bacteriocins produced by Pseudomonas olanacearum. *Annual Phytopathological Society of Japan* 59: 114–122.

9. Aymerich, T., Holo, H., Håvarstein, L. S., Hugas, M., Garriga, M. and Nes, I.F. 1996. Biochemical and genetic characterization of enterocin A from Enterococcus faecium, a new antilisterial bacteriocin in the pediocin family of bacteriocins. *Applied Environmental Microbiology* 62:1676–82.

10. Baumal, R., Musclow, E., Farkas-Himsley, H. and Marks, A. 1982.Variants of an interspecies hybridoma with altered tumorigenicity and protective ability against mouse mycloma tumors. *Cancer Research* 42 (5): 1904–8.

11. Callewaert, R. and De Vuyst, L. 1999. Expanded bed adsorption as a unique unit operation for the isolation of bacteriocins from fermentation media. *Bioseparation* 8: 159–168.

12. Callewaert, R. and De Vuyst, L. 2000. Bacteriocin production with Lactobacillus amylovorus DCE 471 is improved and stabilized by fed-batch fermentation. *Applied Environmental Microbiology* 66: 606–613.

13. Callewaert, R. Holo, H. Devreese, B. Van Beeumen, J., Nes, I. and De Vuyst L.1999. Characterization and production of amylovorin L471, a bacteriocin purified from Lactobacillus amylovorus DCE 471 by a novel three-step method. *Microbiology* 145: 2559–2568.

14. Chen, H. and Hoover, D. G. 2003. Bacteriocins and their Food Applications. *Comprehensive Reviews in Food Science and Food Safety* (2) 82–100.

15. Chen, W. Y. and Echandi, E. 1984. Effects of avirulent bacteriocinproducing strains of Pseudomonas solanacearum on the control of bacterial wilt of tobacco. *Plant Pathology* 33: 245–253.

16. Cintas, L. M., Casaus, P., Fernández, M. F and Hernandez, P.E. 1998. Comparative antimicrobial activity of enterocin L50, pediocin PA-1, nisin A and lactocin S against spoilage and food borne pathogenic bacteria. *Food Microbiology* 15:289–98.

17. Cleveland, J., Montville, T. J., Nes, I. F. and Chikindas, M. L. 2001. Bacteriocins: Safe, natural antimicrobials for food preservation. *International Journal of Food Microbiology* 71:1–20.

18. Cotter, P. D., Hill, C. and Ross, R. P. 2006. What's in a name? Class distinction for bacteriocins. *Nature Reviews Microbiology* 4 (2). Doi: 10.1038/nrmicro1273–c2.

19. Cruz-Chamorro, L., Puertollano, M. A., Puertollano, E., de Cienfuegos, G. A. and de Pablo, M. A. 2006. In vitro biological activities of magainin alone or in combination with nisin. *Peptides* 27 (6): 1201–9. doi:10.1016/j.peptides.2005.11.008. PMID 16356589.

20. de Jong, A., van Hijum, S. A. F. T., Bijlsma, J.J.E., Kok, J. and Kuipers, O. P. 2006. BAGEL: a web-based bacteriocin genome mining tool. *Nucleic Acids Research* 34: W273–W279. doi:10.1093/nar/gkl237. PMID 1538908.

21. de Vos, W. M., Kuipers, O. P., van der Meer, J. R. and Siezen, R. J. 1995. Maturation pathway of nisin and other lantibiotics: post-translationally modified antimicrobial peptides exported by gram positive bacteria. *Molecular Microbiology* 17:427–37.

22. De Vuyst, L. and Vandamme, E. J. 1994. Nisin, an Antibiotic Produced by Lactococcus lactis subsp.Lactis: Properties, Biosynthesis, Fermentation and Applications. In: *Bacteriocins of Lactic Acid Bacteria: Microbiology, Genetics and Applications*. Blackie Academic and Professional, London, England, pp: 151–221.

23. De Vuyst, L. and Leroy, F. 2007. Bacteriocins from Lactic Acid Bacteria: Production, Purification, and Food Applications. *Journal of Molecular Microbiology and Biotechnology* 13:194–199 DOI: 10.1159/000104752.

24. De Vuyst, L., Avonts, L., Hoste, B., Vancanneyt, M., Neysens, P. and Callewaert, R.2004. The lactobin A and amylovorin L471 genes are identical, and their distribution seems to be restricted to the species Lactobacillus amylovorus that is of interest for cereal fermentations. *International Journal of Food Microbiology* 90: 93–106.

25. Desriac, F., Defer, D., Bourgougnon, N., Brillet B., Chevalier, P. L. and Fleury Y. 2010. Bacteriocin as Weapons in the Marine Animal-Associated Bacteria Warfare: Inventory and Potential Applications as an Aquaculture Probiotic. *Marine Drugs* 8: 1153-1177; doe: 10.3390/md8041153.

26. Dhewa T., Pant, S., Goyal, N. and Mishra, V. 2009b. Studies on Adhesive Properties of Food and Fecal Potential Probiotic Lactobacilli. *Journal of Applied Natural Sciences* 1 (2):138–140.

27. Dhewa, T. and Goyal, N. 2009. Effect of Inulin, Honey and Gum Acacia on Growth of Human Faecal Potential Probiotic Lactobacilli. *The ICFAI University Journal of Life Sciences* 3 (3): 29–34.

28. Dhewa, T., Bajpai, V., Pant, S., Saxena, R. K. and Mishra, V. 2010. Antagonistic Activity of Food and Faecal Lactobacilli against common Enteric-pathogens. *Biospectra* (An International Biannual Refereed Life Sciences 4(2) (in press).

29. Dhewa, T., Bajpai, V., Saxena, R.K., Pant, S. and Mishra V. 2009a. Selection of Lactobacillus strains as potential probiotics on basis of in vitro attributes. *International Journal of Probiotics and Prebiotics* 4 (4): XX-XX (In press).

30. Ennahar, S., Sashihara, T., Sonomoto, K. and Ishizaki, A. 2000. Class IIa bacteriocin biosynthesis, structure and activity. *FEMS Microbiology Review* 24: 85-106.

31. Farkas-Himsley, H. and Musclow, C. E. 1986. Bacteriocin receptors on malignant mammalian cells: are they transferrin receptors? *Cell and Molecular Biology* 32 (5): 607–17. PMID 3779762.

32. Farkas-Himsley, H., Freedman, J., Read, S. E, Asad, S. and Kardish, M. 1991. Bacterial proteins cytotoxic to HIV-1-infected cells. *AIDS* 5 (7): 905–7. PMID 1892605.

33. Farkas-Himsley, H., Hill, R., Rosen, B., Arab, S. and Lingwood, C.A. 1995. The bacterial colicin active against tumor cells in vitro and in vivo is verotoxin 1. Proceeding of the National Academy of Sciences U.S.A. 92 (15): 6996–7000. doi:10.1073/pnas.92.15.6996. PMID 7624357.

34. Farkas-Himsley, H. and Yu, H. 1985. Purified colicin as cytotoxic agent of neoplasia: comparative study with crude colicin. *Cytobios* 42 (167-168): 193–207. PMID 3891240.

35. Farkas-Himsley, H. 1980. Bacteriocins—are they broad-spectrum antibiotics? *Journal of Antimicrobial Chemotherapy* 6 (4): 424–6. doi: 10.1093/jac/6.4.424. PMID 7430010.

36. Ferchichi, M., Frère, J. M., Abrouk, K. and Manai, M. 2001. Lactococcin MMFII, a novel class IIa bacteriocin produced by Lactococcus lactis MMFII, isolated from a Tunisian dairy product. *FEMS Microbiology Letters* 205:49–55.

37. Foulquié Moreno, M. R., Leisner, J. J., Tee, L. K., Ley, C., Radu, S., Rusul, G., Vancanneyt, M. and De Vuyst, L. 2002. Microbial analysis of Malaysian tempeh, and characterization of two bacteriocins produced by isolates of Enterococcus faecium. *Journal of Applied Microbiology* 92:147–157.

38. Foulquié Moreno, M. R, Callewaert, R. and De Vuyst, L. 2001. Isolation of bacteriocins through expanded bed adsorption using a hydrophobic interaction medium. *Bioseparation* 10: 45–50.

39. Foulquié Moreno, M. R, Rea, M. C., Cogan, T. M and De Vuyst, L. 2003. Applicability of a bacteriocin producing Enterococcus faecium as a co-culture in Cheddar cheese manufacture. *International Journal of Food Microbiology* 81: 73–84.

40. Frankin, T. J and Snow, G. A. 1975. *Biochemistry of Antimicrobial Action*, 2nd ed. New York: John Wiley and Sons p. 224.

41. Fuller, R. 1989. Probiotics in man and animals. *Journal of Applied Microbiology* 66: 365–378.

42. Georgalaki, M. D., Van den Berghe, E., Kritikos, D., Devreese, B., Van Beeumen, J., Kalantzopoulos, G., De Vuyst, L. and Tsakalidou, E. 2002. Macedocin, a food-grade lantibiotic produced by Streptococcus macedonicus ACA-DC 198. *Applied Environmental Microbiology* 68: 5891–5903.

43. Gratia, A. and Fredericq, P. 1946. *Comptes Rendus des Séances Société de Biologie* 140:1032–1033, Mayr-Harting and others.1972.

44. Gratia, A. 1925. Sur un remarquable example d'antagonisme entre deux souches de colibacille. *Comptes Rendus Société de Biologie* 93: 1040–2.

45. Gratia, J. P. 2000. André Gratia: a forerunner in microbial and viral genetics. Genetics 156 (2): 471–6. PMID 11014798. PMC 1461273.

46. Gravesen, A., Ramnath, M., Rechinger, K. B., Andersen, N., Jansch, L., Hechard, Y., Hastings, J. W. and Knochel, S. 2002. High-level resistance to class IIa bacteriocins is associated with one general mechanism in Listeria monocytogenes. *Microbiology* 148:2361–9.

47. Guder, A., Wiedemann, I. and Sahl, H. G. 2000. Post-translationally modified bacteriocins-the lantibiotics. *Biopolymers* 55:62–73.

48. Hammami, R., Zouhir, A., Ben Hamida, J. and Fliss, I. 2007. BACTIBASE: a new web-accessible database for bacteriocin characterization. *BMC Microbiology* 7: 89. doi:10.1186/1471-2180-7-89. PMID 17941971.

49. Hammami, R., Zouhir, A., Le Lay, C., Ben Hamida, J. and Fliss, I. 2010. BACTIBASE second release: a database and tool platform for bacteriocin characterization. *BMC Microbiology* 10: 22. doi: 10.1186/1471-2180-10-22. PMID 20105292.

50. Hardy, K. G. 1975. Colicinogeny and related phenomena. *Bacteriology Review* 39: 464–515.

51. Hastings, J. W., Sailer, M., Johnson, K., Roy, K. L., Vederas, J. C. and Stiles, M. E. 1991. Characterization of leucocin A-UAL 187 and cloning of the bacteriocin gene from Leuconostoc gelidum. *Journal of Bacteriology* 173:7491–500.

52. Hechard. Y., Derijard, B., Letellier, F. Cenatiempo Y. 1992. Characterization and purification of mesentericin Y105, an anti-Listeria bacteriocin from Leuconostoc mesenteroides. *Journal of General Microbiology* 138:2725–31.

53. Henderson, J. T, Chopko, A. L. and van Wassenaar, P. D. 1992. Purification and primary structure of pediocin PA-1 produced by Pediococcus acidilactici PAC-1.0. *Arch Biochemistry and Biophysics* 295:5–12.

54. Hert, A. P, Roberts, P. D., Momol, M. T., Minsavage, G. V., Tudor-Nelson, S. M. and Jones, J. B. 2005. Relative importance of bacteriocin-like genes in antagonism of Xanthomonas perforans tomato race 3 to Xanthomonas euvesicatoria tomato race 1 strains 259. *Applied Environmental Microbiology* 71: 3581–3588.

55. Heu, S., Oh, J., Kang. Y., Ryu, S., Cho, S. K, Cho, Y. and Cho, M. 2001. gly gene cloning and expression and purification of glycinecin A, a bacteriocin produced by Xanthomonas campestris pv. glycines 8ra. *Applied Environmental Microbiology* 67: 4105–4110.

56. Holck, A. L., Axelsson L, Birkeland S, Aukrust T, Blom, H. 1992. Purification and amino acid sequence of sakacin A, a bacteriocin from Lactobacillus sake Lb706. *Journal of General Microbiology* 138:2715–20.

57. Holtsmark, I., Eijsink, V. G. and Brurberg, M. B. 2008. Bacteriocins from plant pathogenic bacteria. *FEMS Microbiology Letters* 280: 1–7.

58. Hu, F. P. and Young, J. M. 1998. Biocidal activity in plant pathogenic Acidovorax, Burkholderia, Herbaspirillum, Ralstonia and Xanthomonas spp. *Journal of Applied Microbiology* 84: 263–271.

59. Hurst, A. 1981. Nisin. *Advanced Applied Microbiology* 27:85–123.

60. Jack, R. W, Tagg, J. R. and Ray, B. 1995. Bacteriocins of gram-positive bacteria. *Microbiology Review* 59:171–200.

61. Jacob, F., Lwoff, A., Siminovitch, L. and Wallman, E. 1953. Definition de quelques termes relatifs a la Pysogenie. *Ann Institute of Pasteur Paris* 84:222–4.

62. Jimenez-Diaz, R., Ruiz-Barba, J. L., Cathcart, D. P., Holo, H., Nes, I. F., Sletten, K. H. and Warner, P. J. 1995. Purification and partial amino acid sequence of plantaricin S, a bacteriocin produced by Lactobacillus plantarum LPCO10, the activity of which depends on the complementary action of 2 peptides. *Applied Environmental Microbiology* 61:4459–63.

63. Joerger, M. C. and Klaenhammer, T. R. 1986. Characterization and purification of helveticin J and evidence for a chromosomally determined bacteriocin produced by Lactobacillus helveticus 481. *Journal of Bacteriology* 167:439–46.

64. Kellner, R., Jung, G., Horner, T., Zahner, H., Schnell, N., Entian, K, D. and Götz, F. 1988. Gallidermin: a new lanthionine-containing polypeptide antibiotic. *European Journal of Biochemistry* 177:53–9.

65. Klaenhammer, T. R. 1988. Bacteriocins of lactic acid bacteria. *Biochemistry* 70:337–49.

66. Klaenhammer, T. R. 1993. Genetics of bacteriocins produced by lactic acid bacteria. *FEMS Microbiology Review* 12:39–85.

67. Konisky, J. 1982. Colicins and other bacteriocins with established modes of action. *Annual Review of Microbiol* 36:125–44.

68. Lavermicocca, P., Valerio, F., Evidente, A., Lazzaroni, S., Corsetti, A. and Gobbetti, M. 2000. Purification and characterization of novel antifungal compounds from the sourdough Lactobacillus plantarum strain 21B. *Applied Environmental Microbiology* 66: 4084–4090.

69. Leer, R. J., van der Vossen, J. M. B. M., van Giezen, M., van Noort, J. M. and Pouwels, P. H. 1995. Genetic analysis of acidocin B, a novel bacteriocin produced by Lactobacillus acidophilus. *Microbiology* 141:1629-35.

70. Lejeune, R., Callewaert, R., Crabbé, K. and De Vuyst, L. 1998. Modelling the growth and bacteriocin production by Lactobacillus amylovorus DCE 471 in batch cultivation. *Journal Applied Microbiology* 84: 159–168.

71. Leroy, F. and De Vuyst, L. 2000. Sakacins; in Naidu AS (ed.): *Natural Food Antimicrobial Systems*. Boca Raton, CRC Press LLC. pp 589–610.

72. Leroy, F. and De Vuyst, L. 2004. Lactic acid bacteria as functional starter cultures for the food fermentation industry. *Trends in Food Science and Technology* 15: 67–78.

73. Leroy, F. and De Vuyst, L. 1999. Temperature and pH conditions that prevail during the fermentation of sausages are optimal for the production of the antilisterial bacteriocin sakacin K. *Applied Environmental Microbiology* 65: 974–981.

74. Leroy, F. and De Vuyst, L. 2005. Simulation of the effect of sausage ingredients and technology on the functionality of the bacteriocin-producing Lactobacillus sakei CTC 494 strain. *International Journal of Food Microbiology* 100: 141–152.

75. Leroy, F., Verluyten, J. and De Vuyst, L. 2006. Functional meat starter cultures for improved sausage fermentation. *International Journal of Food Microbiology* 106: 270–285.

76. Makras, L., Triantafyllou, V., Fayol-Messaoudi, D., Adriany, T., Zoumpopoulou, G., Tsakalidou, E., Servin, A. and De Vuyst, L. 2006. Kinetic analysis of the antibacterial activity of probiotic lactobacilli towards Salmonella enterica serovars Typhimurium reveals a role for lactic acid and other inhibitory compounds. *Research in Microbiology* 157: 241–247.

77. McAuliffe, O., Ross, R. P. and Hill, C. 2001. Lantibiotics: structure, biosynthesis and mode of action. *FEMS Microbiology Review* 25:285–308.

78. Metivier, A., Pilet, M. F., Dousset, X., Sorokine, O., Anglade, P., Zagorec, M., Piard, J. C., Marion, D., Cenatiempo, Y. and Fremaux, C. 1998. Divercin V41, a new bacteriocin with 2 disulphide bonds produced by Carnobacterium divergens V41: primary structure and genomic organization. *Microbiology* 144: 2837–44.

79. Moll, G. N., Konings, W. N. and Driessen, A. J. M. 1999. Bacteriocins: mechanism of membrane insertion and pore formation. *Antonie Van Leeuwnhoek* 76:185–98.

80. Mørtvedt, C. I., Nissen-Meyer, J., Sletten, K. and Nes, I. F 1991. Purification and amino acid-sequence of lactocin S, a bacteriocin produced by Lactobacillus sake L45. *Applied Environmental Microbiology* 57: 1829–1834.

81. Motlagh, A. M., Bhunia, A. K., Szostek, F., Hansen, T.R., Johnson, M.G. and Ray, B. 1992. Nucleotide and amino acid sequence of pap-gene (pediocin AcH production) in Pediococcus acidilactici H. *Letters in Applied Microbiology* 15:45–8.

82. Musclow, C. E., Farkas-Himsley, H., Weitzman, S. S. and Herridge, M. 1987. Acute lymphoblastic leukemia of childhood monitored by bacteriocin and flowcytometry. *European Journal Cancer and Clinical Oncology* 23 (4): 411–8. doi: 10.1016/0277–5379 (87)90379-8. PMID 3475205.

83. Nes, I. F. and Johnsborg, O. 2004. Exploration of antimicrobial potential in LAB by genomics. *Current Opinion in Biotechnology* 15:100–104.

84. Nes, I. F., Diep, D. B., Havarstein, L. S., Brurberg, M. B., Eijsink, V. and Holo, H. 1996. Biosynthesis of bacteriocins in lactic acid bacteria. *Antonie van Leeuwenhoek* 70:113-28.

85. Nguyen, H. A., Tomita, T., Hirota, M., Kaneko, J., Hayashi, T. and Kamio, Y. 2001. DNA inversion in the tail fiber gene alters the host range specificity of carotovoricin Er, a phage-tail-like bacteriocin of phytopathogenic Erwinia carotovora subsp.carotovora Er. *Journal of Bacteriology* 183: 6274–6281.

86. Nissen-Meyer, J., Holo, H., Håvarstein, L. S., Sletten, K. and Nes, I. F. 1992. A novel lactococcal bacteriocin whose activity depends on the complementary action of 2 peptides. *Journal of Bacteriology* 174:5686–92.

87. Nissen-Meyer, J., Larsen, G. A., Sletten, K., Daeschel, M. and Nes, I. F. 1993. Purification and characterization of plantaricin A, a Lactobacillus plantarum bacteriocin whose activity depends on the action of 2 peptides. *Journal General Microbiology* 139:1973–8.

88. Oresnik, I. J., Twelker, S. and Hynes, M. F. 1999. Cloning and characterization of a Rhizobium leguminosarum gene encoding a bacteriocin with similarities to RTX toxins. *Applied Environmental Microbiology* 65: 2833–2840.

89. Parente, E. and Ricciardi, A. 1999. Production, recovery and purification of bacteriocins from lactic acid bacteria. *Applied Microbiology and Biotechnology* 52:628–38.

90. Parret, A. H., Temmerman, K. and De Mot, R. 2005. Novel lectin-like bacteriocins of biocontrol strain Pseudomonas fluorescens Pf-5. *Applied Environmental Microbiology* 71: 5197–5207.

91. Piard, J. C., Muriana, P. M., Desmazeaud, P. J. and Klaenhammer, T. R. 1992. Purification and partial characterization of lacticin 481, a lanthionine-containing bacteriocin produced by Lactococcus lactis subsp. lactis CNRZ 481. *Applied Environmental Microbiology* 58:279–84.

92. Puniya, A.K., Puniya, M., Nagpal, R., Malik, M., Kumar, S., Mishra V., Dhewa, T., Pant, S. and Singh, K. 2008. Functional dairy Foods: A healthy hope. In: A. Kumar, G. Sahal, and R. P. Kaur (Eds.), *Lecture Notes: Workshop on Biotechnology, Education, Dehradun*: Saraswati Press. pp.195–205.

93. Reeves, P. R. 1972. *The Bacteriocins*. New York: Springer-Verlag. pp.142.

94. Rihakova, J., Belguesmia, Y., Petit, V.W., Pilet, M. F., Prevost, H., Dousset, X. and Drider, D. 2009. Divercin V41 from gene characterization to food applications: 1998–2008, a decade of solved and unsolved questions. *Letters in Applied Microbiology* 48: 1–7.

95. Riley MA. 1998. Molecular mechanisms of bacteriocin evolution. *Annual Review of Genetics* 32:255–78.

96. Sahl, H. G., Jack, R.W. and Bierbaum, G. 1995. Biosynthesis and biological activities of lantibiotics with unique posttranslational modifications. *European Journal of Biochemistry* 230:827–53.

97. Sahl, H. G. and Bierbaum, G. 1998. Lantibiotics: biosynthesis and biological activities of uniquely modified peptides from Gram-positive bacteria. *Annual Review of Microbiology* 52:41–79.

98. Saito, H., Watanabe, T., Osasa, S. and Tado, O. 1979. Susceptibility of normal and tumor cells to mycobacteriocin and mitomycin C. *Hiroshima Journal of Medical Science* 28 (3): 141–6. PMID 521305.

99. Sand, S. L., Haug, T. M., Nissen-Meyer, J. and Sand, O. 2007. The bacterial peptide pheromone plantaricin A permeabilizes cancerous, but not normal, rat pituitary cells and differentiates between the outer and inner membrane leaflet. *Journal of Membrane Biology* 216 (2-3): 61–71. doi: 10.1007/s00232-007-9030-3. PMID 17639368.

100. Schillinger, U., Geisen, R. and Holzapfel, W. H. 1996. Potential of antagonistic microorganisms and bacteriocins for the biological preservation of foods. *Trends in Food Science and Technology* 7:158–64.

101. Schnürer, J. and Magnusson, J. 2005. Antifungal lactic acid bacteria as biopreservatives. Trends in Food Science and Technology 16: 70–78.

102. Strøm, K., Sjøgren, J., Broberg, A. and Schnürer, J.2002. Lactobacillus plantarum MiLAB 393 produces the antifungal cyclic dipeptides cyclo (L - Phe- L - Pro) and cyclo (L-Phe-Trans-4-OH- L - Pro) and 3-phenyllactic acid. *Applied Environmental Microbiology* 68: 4322–4327.

103. Tagg, J. R., Dajani, A. S. and Wannamaker, L. W. 1976. Bacteriocins of gram-positive bacteria. *Bacteriology Review* 40:722–56.

104. Tagg, J.R. and Dierksen, K.P. 2003. Bacterial replacement therapy: adapting 'germ warfare' to infection prevention. *Trends in Biotechnology* 21: 217–223.

105. Tichaczek, P. S., Meyer, J. N., Nes, I. F., Vogel, R. F. and Hammes, W. P.1992. Characterization of the bacteriocins curvacin A from Lactobacillus curvatus LTH1174 and sakacin P from L. sake LTH673. *Systematic Applied Microbiology* 15: 460–468.

106. van Belkum, M. J., Hayema, B. J., Geis, A., Kok, J. and Venema, G. 1991. Organization and nucleotide sequences of 2 lactococcal bacteriocin operons. *Applied Environmental Microbiology* 57:492–8.

107. Van den Berghe, E., Skourtas, G., Tsakalidou, E. and De Vuyst, L. 2006. Streptococcus macedonicus ACA-DC 198 produces the lantibiotic, macedocin, at temperature and pH conditions that prevail during cheese manufacture. *International Journal of Food Microbiology* 107: 138–147.

108. van Kraaij, C., de Vos, W. M., Siezen, R. J., Kuipers, O. P. 1999. Lantibiotics: biosynthesis, mode of action and applications. *Natural Product Reports Articles* 16:575–87.

109. Vaughan, E. E., Daly, C. and Fitzgerald, G. F. 1992. Identification and characterization of helveticin V-1829, a bacteriocin produced by Lactobacillus helveticus 1829. *Journal of Applied Bacteriology* 73:299–308.

110. Venema, K., Venema, G. and Kok, J. 1995. Lactococcal bacteriocins: mode of action and immunity. *Trends in Microbiology* 3:299–304.

111. Wood, B. J. B. and Holzapfel, W. H. 1995. *The Genera of Lactic Acid Bacteria*. London, Blackie Academic and Professional.

112. Worobo, R. W., Henkel, T., Sailer, M., Roy, K. L., Vederas, J. C. and Stiles, M. E. 1994. Characteristics and genetic determinant of a hydrophobic peptide bacteriocin, carnobacteriocin A, produced by Carnobacterium piscicola LV 17A. *Microbiology* 140:517–26.

113. Worobo, R. W., VanBelkum, M. J., Sailer, M., Roy, K. L., Vederas, J. C. and Stiles, M. E. 1995. A signal peptide secretion-dependent bacteriocin from Carnobacterium divergens. *Journal of Bacteriology* 177:3143–9.

114. Yamada, K., Hirota, M., Niimi, Y., Nguyen, H. A., Takahara, Y., Kamio, Y. and Kaneko, J. 2006. Nucleotide sequences and organization of the genes for carotovoricin (Ctv) from Erwinia carotovora indicate that Ctv evolved from the same ancestor as Salmonella typhi prophage. Bioscience *Biotechnology and Biochemistry* 70: 2236–2247.

115. Yang, R., Johnson, M. C. and Ray, B.1992. Novel method to extract large amounts of bacteriocins from lactic acid bacteria. *Applied Environmental Microbiology* 58: 3355–3359.

5

Actinomycetes and Antibiotics: A Review

Garima Arya • Padma Singh

INTRODUCTION

Actinomycetes are best known for their ability to produce antibiotics and are Gram-positive bacteria which comprise a group of branching unicellular microorganisms. They produce branching mycelium which may be of two kind, *viz.* substrate mycelium and aerial mycelium. Among actinomycetes, the *Streptomycetes* are the dominant. Screening of actinomycetes for the production of novel antibiotics has been intensively pursued for many years. Antibiotics have been used in many fields including agriculture, veterinary, and pharmaceutical industry. Actinomycetes have the capability to synthesize many different bioactive secondary metabolites such as antibiotics, herbicides, fungicides, insecticides, pesticides, anti-parasitic and enzymes (Aslan 1999). The discovery of antibiotics had a major impact on the control of infectious diseases and the development of pharmaceutical industry. During the last few decades, the pharmaceutical industry has not only continued to screen microbial metabolites of antimicrobial activity but has successfully extended to the isolation of new compounds for many other medical applications.

Actinomycetes are the major source of bioactive secondary metabolites and representing about 70–80% of all the isolated compounds (Berdy 2005). Actinomycetes like *Streptomyces* form a distinct clad within the radiation encompassed by the high GC Gram-positive bacteria in the 16S rRNA tree. There is an evidence that specific metabolites such as streptomycin, may be synthesized by strains in a specific clad. For example; streptomycin and isolated metabolites appear to be randomly distributed across the whole genome. The specific relationships in the actinomycetes and the way they are reflected in the biosynthetic potential to produce bioactive compounds could significantly influence strategies for search and discovery, screening and bioprocess development (Abraham 1981). Characteristics of the spore bearing hyphae and spore chains

69

(Figs 5.1 to 5.3, colour plate 3) should be determined by using direct microscopic examination of the culture surface. Adequate magnification (400 X) could be used to establish the presence or absence of spore chains and to observe the nature of sporophores.

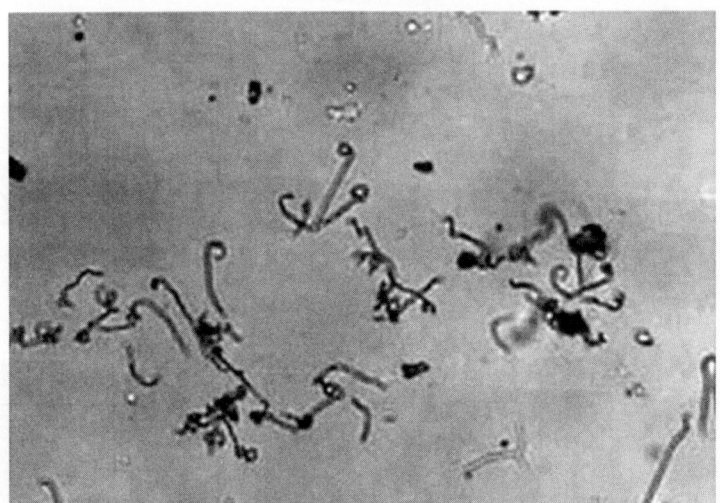

Fig. 5.1: Spiral spore chains (400 X)

Actinomycetes, the Gram-positive, high G + C content filamentous bacteria, are well known as a good source of microbial secondary metabolites producer in antibiotics discovery programs. Many species, especially those belonging to the genus *Streptomyces,* have been studied as potential producers of metabolites with diverse chemical structure and biological activities (Berdy 2005). Ten out of thousands of such compounds are antibiotics used for the treatment of a wide range of diseases infection of human beings. Indeed, the searching for novel actinomycetes constitutes an essential component in natural product-based antibiotics discovery.

The word "antibiotic" is derived from Greek *stems* that means 'against life'. A French researcher Vuillemin coined this term in 1889, when he isolated a substance from *P.* a*eruginosa*. The substance, called pyocyanin, inhibits the growth of other bacteria in the test tubes. Thus "antibiotics are chemical substances produced by certain microorganisms that inhibit or kill another microorganism."

In the last 100 years, there were two periods in which the incidence of disease declined sharply. The first periods took place in the early 1900s. At this time, an understanding of the disease process led to numerous social measures such as water putrification, careful food production, insect control, milk pasteurization and patient isolation. Sanitary practices made it possible to prevent virulent microorganisms from reaching their human targets. The second period began in 1940s with the development of antibiotics, and blossomed in the years thereafter when physicians found that they could treat established cases of disease, major were made as serious illnesses came under control.

About 50 years ago, antibiotics were introduced for the treatment of microbial diseases. Since then, the greatest threat to the use of antimicrobial agents for therapy of bacterial

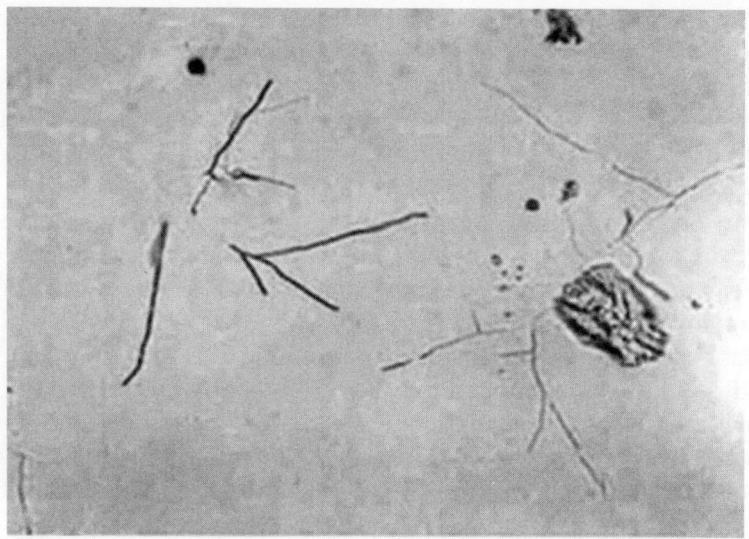

Fig. 5.2: RF spore chains (400 X)

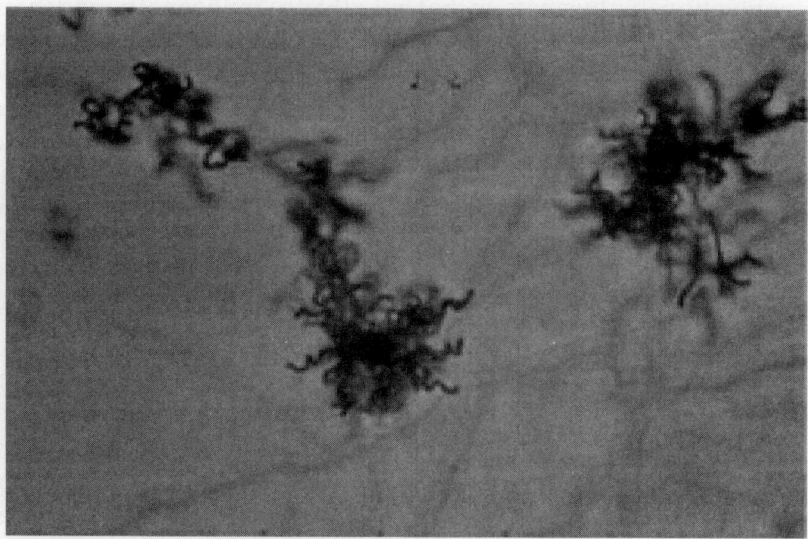

Fig. 5.3: RA spore chains (400 X)

infections has been the development of antimicrobial resistance in pathogenic bacteria. Antibiotic resistance has been shown to have occurred rarely in bacteria collected before the antibiotic era. Shortly after the introduction of each new antimicrobial compound, emergence of antimicrobial resistance is observed (Levy, 1997). The magnitude of the problem is significantly increased by the possibility of bacteria to transfer resistance determinants horizontally and by the mounting increase in the use (over-use and misuse) of antibiotics, which has created an enormous selective pressure towards resistant bacteria (Levy, 1992). Prescott (2002) concluded that gene transfer occurs widely in vivo between gastrointestinal tract bacteria and pathogenic bacteria, as identical resistance genes are present in diverse bacterial species from different hosts. In fact, we face the frightening probability that most pathogenic bacteria that threaten human health will soon be resistant to all known antibiotics. However, for several decades, studies on the selection and dissemination of antibiotic resistance have focused mainly on clinically relevant bacterial species.

The evolution of antibiotic resistant food-borne pathogens has been amply documented in recent years. Recently, many investigators have speculated that commensal bacteria may act as reservoirs of antibiotic resistance genes similar to those found in human pathogens (Igrashi et al 1955, Levy and Salyers, 2002) and are thus very important in our understanding of how antibiotic resistance genes are maintained and spread through bacterial populations (Levy 2004 and Miller, 1989). The main threat associated with these bacteria is that they can transfer resistance genes to pathogenic bacteria. Such reservoir organisms could possibly be found in various foods and food products containing high densities of non-pathogenic bacteria as a result of their natural production process.

Economic Importance of Antibiotics

The sale of antibiotics is big business. In the United States, millions of pounds of antibiotics valued at billions of dollars are produced annually. Approximately, 40 to 50% of these antibiotics are added to livestock feed. Because of the massive quantities of antibiotics being prepared and used, an increasing number of diseases are resisting treatment due to the spread of drug resistance. A good example is *Neisseria gonorrhoeae*, the causative agent of gonorrhea. Gonorrhea was first treated successfully with sulphonamide in 1936, but in 1945 most strains were resistant and physicians turned to penicillin. Within 16 years, a penicillin-resistant strain had emerged in the fast test. A penicillinase producing gonococcus reached the United States in 1976 and is still spreading in this country.

A very large number of antibiotics have been discovered, but less than 1% have been of practical value in medicine. However, the useful antibiotics have a dramatic impact on the treatment of infectious disease. Further, many antibiotics are made more effective by chemical modifications in the laboratory; these are said to be semisynthetic antibiotics.

One of the first to postulate the existence and value of antibiotics was the British microbiologist Alexander Fleming. In 1928, who was performing research on *Staphylococci* on to plates of nutrient agar, he noted that one plate was contaminated by a green mould. His interest was piqued by the failure of *Staphylococci* to grow near the mould. Fleming isolated the mould identified it as a species of *Penicillium* and Gram-positive bacteria. Although he failed to isolate the elusive substance, he named it penicillin.

Production of Antibiotics by Actinomycetes

The isolation of streptomycin was the culminating point of a painstaking search for antimicrobial agents produced by actinomycetes, a group of organisms closely related to the bacteria. This was preceded by long and continuous research, dating back to 1915, on actinomycetes, their occurrence of streptomycin 373 and abundance in nature, their systematic or taxonomic position, their role in soil processes, notably in the decomposition of plant and animal residues and in the formation of humus, and finally their associative and antagonistic effects upon bacteria and fungi. It was finally established that as many as 20 to 50% of all the actinomycetes found in the soil and in other natural substrates had the capacity to inhibit the growth of other microorganisms. According to Waksmann 1949, 57, 62, *Streptomyces griseus*, the organism which comprised the streptomycin producing strain, was known in our laboratories from the beginning of our work on actinomycetes, although it was not tested at that time for its antibiotic-producing properties. The ability of actinomycetes to exert injurious effects upon bacteria and fungi has been known for many years and abundance in nature, their systematic or taxonomic position, their role in soil processes, notably in the decomposition of plant and animal residues and in the formation of humus, and finally their associative and antagonistic effects upon bacteria and fungi. It was finally established that as many as 20 to 50 per cent of all the actinomycetes found in the soil and in other natural substrates had the capacity to inhibit the growth of other microorganisms cultures of organisms designated as *Streptothrix*, and now known to be actinomycetes, are capable of dissolving living and dead bacterial cells. The first survey of the occurrence of antagonistic actinomycetes in the soil: 80 cultures were isolated, of which 47 were able to repress bacterial growth, but only 27 liberated into the medium substances which had the capacity to inhibit the growth of Gram-positive bacteria, but not of Gram-negative bacteria or fungi.

Waksmann (1957) also said in his lecture that began his investigation on the production of antibiotics by actinomycetes in 1939, only two preparations were known to possess antimicrobial properties. These were not true antibiotics, or at least were not recognized as such. One was obtained by Gratia and had the capacity to lyse dead typhoid cells and certain living bacteria; it was later designated by Welsch as actinomycetin. The other was believed to be a lysozyme, which had lytic principles, and was studied by Krassilnikov and Koreniako in 1939. The first true antibiotic to be derived from a culture of an actinomyces was isolated in 1940. The organism, *Actinomyces antibioticus*, yielded a substance which was designated as actinomycin. It was soon crystallized, and its chemical and biological properties were established. This antibiotic proved to be a quinone-like pigment with an approximate molecular formula of $C_{41}H_{56}N_8O_{11}$. It was highly active against various Gram-positive bacteria but to a much lesser degree upon the Gram-negative organisms. It proved to be extremely toxic to experimental animals species. Some organisms give rise to different modifications of the same antibiotic, as actinomycin A, B, and C. This is true also of streptomycin, various modifications of which are produced by different species of *Streptomyces*, notably *S. griseus*, *S. bikiniensis*, and *S. griseocarneus* (streptomycin, mannosidostreptomycin, hydroxystreptomycin). Some organisms produce a mixture of different antibiotics, as in the case of different strains of *S. griseus*, which give rise not only to streptomycin, but also to the antifungal agents actidone and candicin (Table 5.1). The various infectious diseases have been divided, in their relation to streptomycin, as follows.

Disease Definitely Indicated for Actinomycetes Producing Antibiotics Treatment

1. All cases of tularemia.

2. All cases of *H. influenzae* infections:
- Meningitis
- Endocarditis
- Laryngotracheitis
- Urinary tract infections
- Pulmonary infections

3. All cases of meningitis due to:
- *E. coli*
- *Pr. vulgaris*
- *K. pneumoniae*
- *B. lactis-aerogenes*
- *Ps. aeruginosa*
- *S. paratyphi*

4. All cases of bacteremia due to Gram-negative organisms:
- *E. coli*
- *Pr. vulgaris*
- *A. aerogenes*
- *Ps. aeruginosa*
- *K. pneumoniae*

5. Urinary tract infections due to:
- *E. coli*
- *Pr. vulgaris*
- *K. pneumoniae*
- *B. lactis-aerogenes*
- *II. influenzae*
- *Ps. aeruginosa*

Table 5.1: Antibiotics produced by major group of microorganisms

Taxonomic group	Number of antibiotics
Bacteria other than actinomycetes	950
Actinomycetes	4600
Fungi	1600

Worldwide antibiotics production is over 10,000 tons/year and estimated gross scale for 1980 were $ 4.2 billion. The annual gross scale in the United State alone is 1 billion, the feed additive antibiotics are believed to have a world market of $ 100 million annually.

Microorganisms as a Source of Antibiotics

Fleming was not the first to note the antibacterial qualities of *Penicillium* species, Joseph Lister had observed a similar phenomenon in 1871; John Tyndall did like wise in 1876.

In same time, Florey, a pathologist and Chain, biochemist has reisolated Fleming's penicillin. Physiology or medicine in 1945 for the discovery and development of penicillin. In the late 1950s, the beta-lactam nucleus of the penicillin molecule was identified and synthesized, the scientist found they could attach various groups to this nucleus and create new penicillins. In the following years, thousands of penicillins emerged from this semisynthetie process.

Ampicillin exemplifies a semisynthetic penicillin. It is less active against Gram-positive cocci then penicillin G. Amoxicillin, a chemical relative of ampicillin. Carbenicillin, methicillin, natcillin, piperacillin, oxacillin, and ticarcillin (combined with claceulanic acid, combination of both known as timentin), etc. are developed. Streptomycin is basically hydrochloride of streptomycin with calcium chloride streptomycin discovered by Gordoh (1966), Burgei (1993) and Wakslman (1949, 62) who were researcher at Rutgers University isolated from the mold-like bacterium *S. griseus*. In this, an Italian microbiologist observed a striking difference in the amount of *E.coli* in two adjoining areas. Subsequently, he discovered a fungus *Cephalosporium acremonium*, which was producing an antibacterial substance in water. The substance named cephalosporin C, later on the basis of call rises of antibiotics its known as cephalosporin. Neomycin and kanamycin are two older antibiotics of the aminoglycoside group, having been isolated from *Streptomyces* sp. in 1949 and 1957, respectively.

Discovery of chloramphenicol in 1947 was a milestone in microbiology. Because chloramphenicol is a broadspectrum antibiotic. The scientists of Ledererly laboratories discovered first tetracycline antibiotic in 1948. In the 1970, researchers discovered erythromycin. Monobactams are a group of antibiotics first synthesized by researchers at Squibb laboratories in the early 1980. Physicians, professor and writer; one of his notable books is a collection of essays entitled "The Youngest Science: Notes of a Medicine – Watcher (1983)". The ability to synthesize antibiotics are reviewed. There are relatively some reports concerning antibiotics production by actinomycetes. Many also tend to be dated as can be seen from Table 5.2.

Indeed, different *Streptomyces* species produce about 75% of commercially and medically useful antibiotics. They have provided more than half of the naturally occurring antibiotics discovered to date and continue to be screened for useful compounds (Miyadoh 1993). Search for new antibiotics effective against multi-drug resistant pathogenic bacteria is presently an important area of antibiotic research. Natural products having novel structures have been observed to possess useful biological activities. Soil is a natural reservoir for microorganisms and their antimicrobial products (Dancer 2004). Filamentous soil bacteria belonging to the genus *Streptomyces* are widely recognized as industrially important microorganisms because of their ability to produce many kinds of novel secondary metabolites including antibiotics (Williams et al. 1965, Crandall and Hamil 1986, Williams et al. 1983 and Korn 1992). Of all known drugs, 70% have been isolated from actinomycetes bacteria of which 75% and 60% are used in medicine and agriculture, respectively (Miyadoh 1993).

Mode of Antimicrobial Agent

There are four major locations of actions of antimicrobioal agent:
1. Inhibition of synthesis of cell wall peptidoglycan. Antimicrobial agent— cephalosporin, vancomycin, etc.
2. Damage of permeability to the cytoplasmic membrane —gentamicin, polymycin, etc.
3. Inhibition of protein synthesis, e.g. streptomycin and chloramphenicol.
4. Inhibition of nucleic acid synthesis, e.g. rifamycin.

Table 5.2: Some antibiotics produced by actinomycetes

Antibiotics	Producing actinomycetes
Actinomycin	*Actinomyces* sp.
Chloramphenicol	*S. venezuelae*
Cycloheximide	*S. griseus*
Cycloserine	*S. orchidaceus*
Erythromycin	*S. erythreus*
Kanamycin	*S. kanamyceticus*
Linkomycin	*S. lincolnensis*
Micromonosporin	*Micromonospora* sp.
Neomycin	*S. fradiae*
Nystatin	*S. noursei*
Rifamycin	*Streptomyces* sp.
Streptomycin	*S. griseus*
Tetracyclin	*S. rimosus*
Neomycin	*S. fradiae*
Granaticin	*S. thermovialaceous*
Thermomycin	*S. thermophillus*
Thermorobin	*T. antibioticus*
T-SA-125	*Thermonospora* sp.
Thermoviridin	*Thermoactinomyces viridis*
Thermothiocin	*Thermoactinopolyspora cormialis*

It is crucial to recognize that the antibiotic therapy is not a simple matter. Antibiotics may be administrated in several different ways and they do not spread rapidly throughout the body or immediately kill all invading pathogens. A complex array of factor influence the effectiveness of antibiotics. The antimicrobial agent can damage pathogens in several ways, as can be seen in Table 5.3.

The discovery of novel antibiotics and non-antibiotics molecules of pharmaceutical interest through microbial secondary metabolites screening is becoming increasingly fruitful. There is a wide acceptance that microorganisms are virtually unlimited source of novel structures with many therapeutic applications. Actinomycetes, among them hold a prominent position due to their diversity and proven ability to produce new structure. It is possible to use special isolation media for enrichment of desired microorganism. Selective isolation is based on condition (s) which favour the growth or survival of the desired microorganism and reduce or eliminate the unwanted growth. One wants to isolate organisms belonging to particular genera or may be interested in actinomycetes which produce antibacterial or antifungal agents and that only depends on media or strains.

During the past 25 years, an alarming number of bacterial strains have evolved with resistance to chemotherapeutic agent and antibiotics. In 1997, an MRSA strain evolved intermediate vancomycin resistance, scientist named it VIRSA, for vamcomycin intermediately resistant *Staphylococcus aureus*. Scientist may show us how to avoid infectious microorganisms and doctors may be able to control certain diseases with antibiotics, but the ultimate body defence depends upon the immune system and other natural measure of resistance. The antibiotics supplement natural defences, they do not replace them.

Table 5.3: Mechanisms of action of antimicrobial agent

Antimicrobial agent	Mechenism of action
Cell wall synthesis inhibition	
Penicillin	Inhibits transpeptidation enzymes envoloved in cross-
Ampicillin	linking of the polysaccharide chains of bacterial cellwall Peptidoglycan. Activate cell wall lytic enzymes.
Carbenicillin	
Methicillin	
Cephalosporins	
Vancomycin	Binds to D-ala terminus and inhibits transpeptidation
Bacitracin	Inhibits cell wall synthesis.
Protein synthesis inhibition	
Streptomycin	Binds with 30 S subunit of the bacterial ribosome to inhibit
Gentamicin	protein synthesis.
Chloramphenicol	Binds to the 50 S ribosomal subunit and blocks peptide bond formation through inhibition of peptidyl transferase.
Tetracycline	Binds to 30 S rRNA and interferes with aminoacyl-t RNA.
Erythromycin	Binds to the 50 S rRNA and inhibits peptide chain
Clindamycin	elongation.
Fusidic acid	Bind to EF-G and blocks translocation.
Nucleic acid synthesis inhibition	
Ciprofloxacin	Inhibits bacterial DNA gyrase and thus interferes with DNA
Quinolones	Replication, transcription and other activity involving DNA.
Rifamycin	Blocks RNA synthesis by binding and inhibiting DNA-dependent RNA polymerase.
Cell membrane disruption	
Polymyxin B	Binds to plasma membrane and disrupts its structure and permeability properties.
Metabolic antagonism	
Sulfonamide	Inhibits folic acid synthesis.
Trimethoprim	Blocks tetrahydrofolate synthesis through dihydrofolate reductase enzymes.
Dapsone	Interfers with folic acid synthesis.

Conclusion

Antibiotics have traditionally been known as miracle drugs, but there is growing body of evidence that are becoming over worked miracles. Some researchers suggest that antibiotic should be controlled as strictly as narcotics. The antibiotic roulette that is currently taking place should be a matter of discussion for all individuals concerned about infectious diseases, be they scientist or student.

REFERENCES

1. Aslan B. 199. Studies on isolation, characterization and antibiotic production of *Streptomyces* species. PhD thesis, Cukurova University, Institute of Science, Adana.
2. Abraham E P. 1981. The beta-lactum antibiotics. *Sci. Am.* 244(6):76–86.
3. Berdy J. 2005. Bioactive microbial metabolites. A personal view. *J. Antibiot.*
4. Bevan P, Ryder H. 1995. Show I. Identify small molecular lead compounds: The screening approach to drug discovery. *Biotechnol.*, 113: 115–121.
5. Burgei CE, Montgomery JA. 1993. Drugs by design. *Sci. Am.* 269(6):92–98.
6. Casida, L.E. 1997. Fermentation: Antibiotics production and other industrial methods. *Industrial Microbiology*, New age International Publisher, 9th edition. pp. 51–250.
7. Crandall, L.W., Hamil, R.L., 1986. Antibiotics produced by *Streptomyces*: major structural classes. In: Queener SW, Day LE (eds), *The bacteria*, Vol. 9, Academic Press, Orlando, Fla, 355–401.
8. Dancer, S.J., 2004. How antibiotics can make us sick: the less obvious adverse effects of antimicrobial chemotherapy. *The Lancet Infectious Diseases* 4, 611–619.
9. Drautz, H., H. Zaehner, J. Rohr and A. Zeeck, 1986. *Journal of Systematic Bacteriology*, 24: 54–63. Metabolic products of microorganisms. Urdamycins.
10. Dietz, A., 1994. The lives and times of industrial actinomycetes. *ASM News* 60: 366–369.
11. Gordon, R.E., 1966. Some criteria for the recognition new angucycline antibiotics from *Streptomyces frdiae*. *Isolation, Characterization and Biological Microbiology*, 45: 355–364.
12. Hopwood, D.A., and Merrick, M.J., 1977. Genetics of antibiotics production. *Bacterilogical Review Sept.* 595–635.
13. Hyakaw, M., Ishizawa, K., Yamazaki, T., and Nohomura,H.,1995. Distribution of antibiotic producing microbiospora strain...... 75–79.
14. Igarashi, M., Kinoshita, N., Ikeda, T., Kameda, M., and Takeuchi,T., 1997. Resormycin, a novel herbicide and antifungal antibiotics produced by a strain of *Streptomyces plantensis*, *Journal of Antibiotics*, Tokyo. 1020–1025.
15. Igarashi, M., K. Ogata and A. Miyake, 1955. *Streptomyces*: Fradicin-mycelin group substance. J. Antibiot, pp: 113–117.*World Appl. Sci. J.*, 6 (11): 1495–1505,
16. Korn, W. F., and Kutzner, H.J., 1992. The family Streptomycetaceae. In: Balows A, Truper HG, Dworkin M, Harder W, Schleifer KH (eds), *The prokaryotes*, Springer-Verlag, New York, 921–995.
17. Lechevalier, H.A., 1989. The actinomycetes ill, a practical guide to generic identification of Actinomycetes. *Bergey's Manual of Systematic Bacteriology*, Vol. 4, Williams and Wilkins Company, Baltimore, 2344–2347.
18. Levy, S.B., 2002. *The Antibiotic Paradox: How Misuse of Antibiotics Destroys their Curative Powers*. 2nd (ed), Perseus Books, Boston.
19. Levy, S.B., and Marshall, B., 2004. Antibacterial resistance worldwide: causes, challenges and responses. *Nature Medicine* 10, 122–129.
20. Livornese LL Jr, Slavin D, Gilbert B, Robbins P, Santoro J. Use of antibac-terial agents in renal failure. *Infect Dis Clin North Am* 2004; 18:551–79.
21. Madigan, M.T., Martinco, J.M., and Jack, M., Antibiotic production. *Brock Biology of Microorganisms*, Prentice Hall International Inc. 8th edi. 392–398.
22. Miyadoh, S., 1993. Research on antibiotic screening in Japan over the last decade: A producing microorganisms approach. *Actinomycetologica* 9, 100–106.
23. Miller, R.M., 1969. *Phosphonomycin. Discovery and Cambridge*, Univ. Press. *in vitro* biological characterization. *Antimicr. Agents* 21.
24. Jones, K., 1949. Fresh isolates of actinomycetes. *Chemother*, pp: 284–290.

25. Matsushima, R.G., Baltz, R.H., Seno, J., Stonesifer P. Matsushima R.G. Benedict, 1957. A section of media for and G.M. Wild, 1981.Genetics and biochemistry of maintenance and taxonomic study of *Streptomycetes.* tylosin production by *Streptomyces fradiae. Antibiotics Ann.,* pp: 947–953. pp: 371–375. *In* D. Schelesinger (ed.). 23. Gordon, R.E., D.A. Barnett, J.E. Handehan .

26. Prescott, L.M., Harley, J.P., and Klein, D.A., 2002. *Microbiology: Antimicrobial Chemotherapy.* 4th edi. Mc-Graw Hill.677–696.

27. Stapley, E.O., Hendlin, M.J., Martinez, M. J., Cowan, S.T., 1974. Cowan and Steel's Manual for H. Wallick, S. Hernandez, S. Mochales, S. Currie and The Identification of Medical Bacteria.

28. Shirilling, E.B. and D. Gottlieb, 1966. Methods for actinomycetes in soil. *J. Gen. Microbiol.,* 38: 251–262.

29. S. A. Waksman, *Streptomycin, its Nature and Practical Application,* Williams andWilkins Co., Baltimore, Md., 1949.

30. Williams, S.T. and F.L. Davies, 1965. Use of Bacteriology, 20: 435–443. antibiotics for selective isolation and enumeration of actinomycetes in soil. *J. Gen. Microbiol.,* 38: 251–262

31. Waksman, S.A., and Lechevalier, H.A., 1957. Chapman, G.S., 1952. A simple method for making Neomycin Rutgers Research and Eucational multiple tests on a microorganism. *J. Bacteriol.,* Foundation. US Patent 2799620 19570716. 63: 147.

32. Waksman, S.A., and H.A., Lechevalier, 1962. Hankin, L., M. Zucker and D.C. Sands, 1971. Description of antibiotics. pp. 206–307. *In* The Improved solid medium for the detection andActinomycetes vol III: Antibiotics of Actinomycetes. enumeralion of proteolytic bacteria. *Appl. Microbiol.,* The Williams and Wilkins Company, Baltimore. 22: 205–509.

33. Williams, S.T., Goodfellow, M., Alderson. G., Wellington, E.M.H., Sneath, P.H.A., and Sackin, M.J.1983. Numerical classification of *Streptomyces* and related genera. *Journal of General Microbiology* 129, 1743–1813.

6

Medicinal Importance of Spices of Umbelliferae

Surbhi Kaushik • Padma Singh

INTRODUCTION

Apiaceae or Umbelliferae is a family of usually aromatic plants with hollow stems, commonly known as umbellifers. It includes cumin, parsley, anise, carrot, coriander/cilantro, dill, caraway, fennel, parsnip, celery, etc. It is a large family with about 300 genera and more than 3,000 species. The earlier name Umbelliferae derives from the inflorescence being generally in the form of a compound "umbel", and has the same root as the word "umbrella". Many members of this plant group are cultivated for various purposes. Plants of this category also are adapted to conditions that encourage heavy concentrations of essential oils, so that some are used as flavorful or aromatic herbs, such as parsley, cilantro, and dill. The plentiful seeds of the umbers, likewise, are sometimes used in cuisine, as with coriander, fennel, cumin, and caraway. Plant derived products have been used for medicinal purposes for centuries.

Significance of the Spices and Herbal Drugs

At present, it is estimated that about 80% of the world population rely on botanical preparations as medicines to meet their health needs. Herbs and spices are generally considered safe and proved to be effective against certain ailments. They are also extensively used, particularly, in many Asian, African and other countries. In recent years, in view of their beneficial effects, use of spices/herbs has been gradually increasing in developed countries also. Many plants and their products have antimicrobial substances that are formed in nature to protect them against spoilage due to microorganisms. These substances save human beings and other animals from diseases. Despite modern medical practice with its high tech methods and synthesised drugs and remedies, many people still hold to more traditional methods of treatments and cures using commonly obtainable herbs and spices. Every spice, every herb, every plant from black pepper seeds through cinnamon to mango, banana and foxglove may be used in the practice of alternative medicine (Fig. 6.1, colour plate 3).

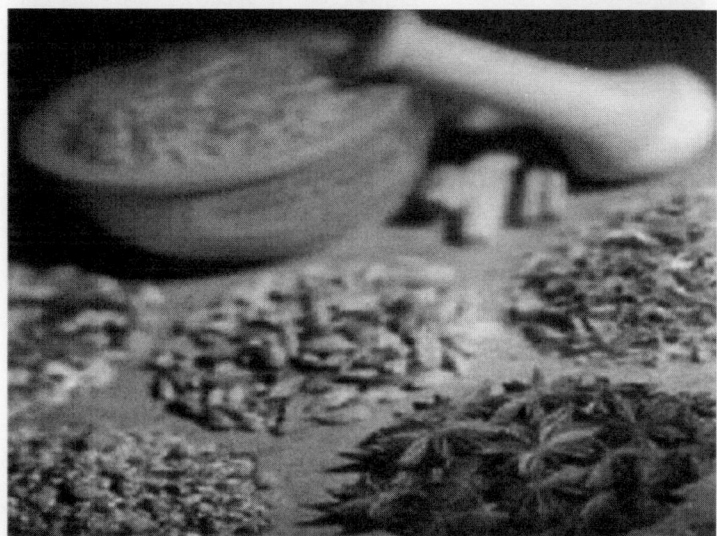

Fig. 6.1: Different spices used as alternative medicine throughout the world

Natural products have played an important role throughout the world in treating and preventing human diseases. Natural product medicines have come from various source materials including terrestrial plants, terrestrial microorganisms, marine organisms, and terrestrial vertebrates and invertebrates (Newman *et al.* 2000).

The search of antibiotics (i.e. secondary metabolites having pharmaceutical values and produced by microorganism such as bacteria, actinomycetes and fungi during their stationary phase of growth) began in the late 1800s.

Alexander Fleming, a Scottish physician and bacteriologist, almost tossed out some plates that had been contaminated by mould. Fortunately, he took a second look at the curious pattern of growth on the contaminated plates. There was a clear area around the mould where the bacterial culture had stopped growing. Fleming was looking at a mold that was later identified as *Penicillium notatum* and in 1928 Fleming named the mold's active inhibitor *penicillin* and discovered first antibiotic. Thus, penicillin is an antibiotic produced by a fungus (Prescott *et al.* 2005). During that time, Fleming warned that the misuse of penicillin could lead to the emergence of resistant forms of bacteria (Fig. 6.2, colour plate 4).

In India, over 2600 plants species have been considered useful in the traditional system of medicine like Ayurveda, Unani, Siddha and home remedies. The drugs that were used thousand of years ago are being employed today also to cure some types of diseases (Ambasta, 1986). The Rig Veda, perhaps the oldest repositories of human knowledge having been written about 4500–1600 BC claims about 99 medicinal plants. Atharva Veda deals with 288 plants (129 according to Dr Udupa), almost all have medicinal ingredients and were used to cure deadly diseases (Kaushik and Dhiman, 2000).

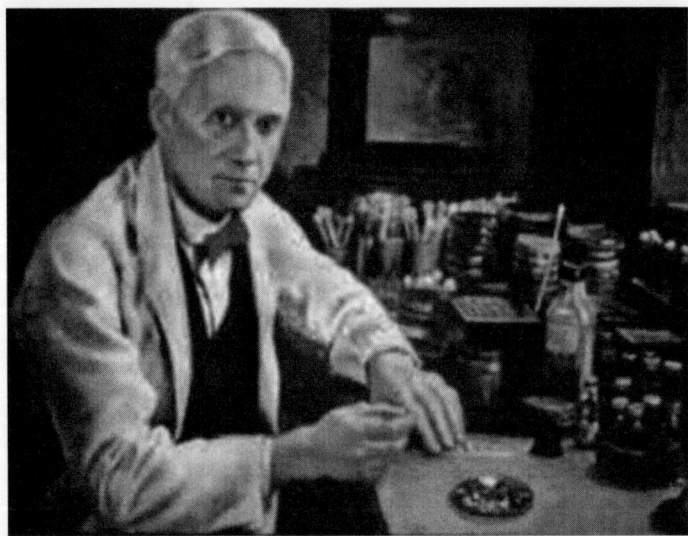

Fig. 6.2: Alexander Fleming, working in his laboratory

A number of Indian scientists have done work in the field of screening of Indian plants for biological activity (Aswal *et al*. 1984). However, a little information is available on the scientific data indicating antimicrobial activity of Ayurvedic drugs (Patel *et al*. 1984, Bhakuni *et al*. 1969).

Properties of Spices

Spice with strong and pungent flavours has been used in the past not only in cookery, but also for preserving food before the advert of refrigeration. The medicinal plants are excellent source of new drug agents which form a basis for the treatment of disease in both traditional and modern medicines and they continue to play a crucial role in the primary health care of many cultures (Fransworth *et al*. 1985). For centuries, medicinal plants have been used all over the world for the treatment and prevention of various ailments, particularly in developing countries where infectious diseases are endemic and modern health facilities are inadequate. Elsewhere, many potent drugs have been purified from medicinal plants including antimalarial, anticancer, anti-diabetic and antibacterial compounds (Samine *et al*. 2005).

Detail of Different Spices

During the middle ages, spices were considered important medicine, but today relatively few are to be found in official drug and used primarily for imparting a pleasant taste to otherwise disagreeable medicines. A few have antiseptic and carminative properties. Apart from their culinary uses, spices are used as flavouring agents in beverages, as active ingredients in ayurvedic medicine, as colouring agents for textiles and as important constituents in cosmetics and perfumery products. Spices stimulate the appetite and increase the flow of gastric juices and for this reason they are often termed as food "accessories" or "adjuncts". They increase the rate of perspiration, thus having a cooling effect on the body. The flavoring, preservative and antiseptic properties of some of these spices are primarily due to the presence of volatile oils, but are occasionally due to other aromatic substances such as alkaloids as in pepper. Some important spices are described below:

Cuminum Cyminum

Vernacular names: Eng: Cumin; Hindi: Zeera

Description: Cumin is the seed of a small umbelliferous plant. The seeds come as paired or separate carpels, and are 3–6 mm (1/8–1/4 in) long. They have a striped pattern of nine ridges and oil canals, and are hairy, brownish in colour, boat-shaped, tapering at each extremity, with tiny stalks attached. They are available dried, or ground to a brownish-green powder. It has a spicy-sweet aroma with pungent, powerful, sharp and slightly bitter flavour (Fig. 6.3, colour plate 4).

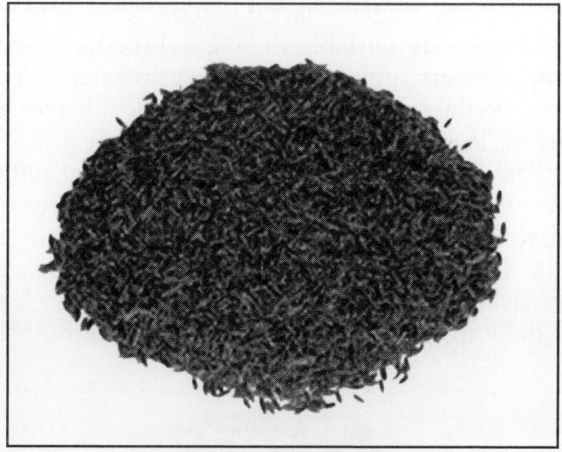

Fig. 6.3: Cumin seeds

Chemical composition: The strong aromatic smell and warm, bitter taste of Cumin fruits are due to the presence of a volatile oil, cumin aldehyde, which exists in the proportion 2.5 to 4%. It is separated by distillation of the fruit with water. It is limpid and pale yellow in colour, and is mainly a mixture of cymol or cymene and cuminic aldehyde, or cyminol, which is its chief constituent.

The main components of *C. cyminum* oil are p-mentha-1,4-dien-7-al, cumin aldehyde, gamma-terpinene, and beta-pinene, (Lacobellis *et al.* 2005). Besides the essential oil, the seeds contain around 10% of the fixed oil. In toasted cumin fruits, a large number of pyrazines has been identified as flavour compounds. Besides pyrazine and various alkyl derivatives (particularly, 2, 5- and 2, 6-dimethyl pyrazine), 2-alkoxy-3-alkylpyrazines seem to be the key compounds (2-ethoxy-3-isopropyl pyrazine, 2-methoxy-3-*sec*-butyl pyrazine, 2-methoxy-3-methyl pyrazine). Also a sulfur compound, 2-methylthio-3-isopropyl pyrazine, was found. All these Maillard-products are also formed, when fenugreek and coriander are toasted.

Medicinal uses: As a medicinal plant, cumin has been utilized as a stimulant, antispasmodic, carminative and sedative. Cumin oil has been reported to have antibacterial activity. *C. cyminum* is a potent immunomodulator and may develop as a lead to recover the immunity of immuno-compromised individuals, (Chauhan *et al.* 2010). It is used as a corrective for the flatulency of languid digestion and as a remedy for colic and dyspeptic headache. It was recommended as a cure for stitches and pains in the side caused by the sluggish congestion of indolent parts. Its principal employment is in veterinary medicine. Bay-salt and Cumin-seeds mixed, is a universal remedy for the diseases of pigeons, especially scabby backs and breasts.

Coriander Sativum

Vernacular names: Sans: Dhanyaka; Hindi: Dhaniya; Beng: Dhane; Tam: Kothamalli; Eng: Coriander

Description: It is an annual, soft, hairless, foetid plant growing to 1 to 3 feet high with erect stems which are slender and branched. It is a bright green, shining, globrous plant. The bright, green leaves are fan-shaped and become more feathery towards the top of the plant. The leaves are variable in shape, broadly lobed at the base of the plant, and slender and feathery higher on the flowering stems. The lowest leaves are stalked and pinnate while the segments of the uppermost leaves are linear and finely divided into very narrow, lacy segments. The flowers are borne in small, shortly-stalked umbels, white or very pale pink, five to ten rays, asymmetrical, with the petals pointing away from the center of the umbel longer than those pointing to the middle of the umbel. The seed clusters are very symmetrical and the seeds fall as soon as ripe (Fig. 6.4, colour plate 4). The fruits are globular dry schizocarp brown to yellow, 3–5 mm diameter, consist of two, single-seeded mericarps. They lose their disagreeable scent on drying and the longer they are kept, the more fragrant they become.

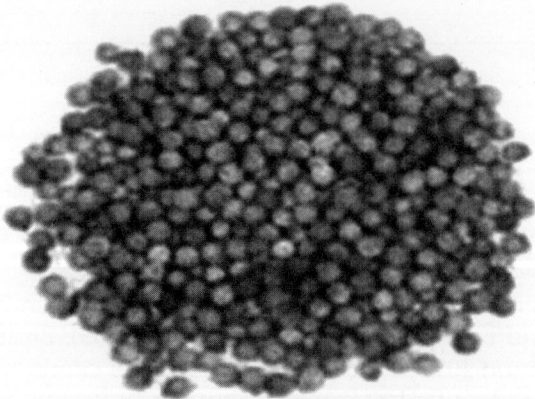

Fig. 6.4: Coriander seeds

Chemical composition: Coriander fruit contains about 1% of volatile oil, which is the active ingredient. It is pale yellow or colourless, and has the odour of Coriander and a mild aromatic taste. It also contains malic acid, tannin and some fatty matter. It has a lemony citrus flavour, when crushed, due to the presence of the terpenes linalool and pinene. Its fruit contains watery content which is about 11.2%. It contains protein which is 14.1%, fatty acid 16.1%, carbohydrate 21.6%, and minerals 44%. The active ingredient in the coriander is essential oil named coriandrol is about 45 to 70%. Coriander essential oil is used as a flavour ingredient, but it also has a long history as a traditional medicine. It is obtained by steam distillation of the dried fully ripe fruits (seeds) of *Coriandrum sativum* L. The oil is a colourless or pale yellow liquid with a characteristic odour and mild, sweet, warm and aromatic flavour, linalool is the major constituent (around 70%) (George *et al.* 2009).

Medicinal Uses

Coriander is used to treat digestive ailments. It is a carminative and used for windy colic. It is stimulant, aromatic and carminative diuretic, stomachic, refrigerant, aphrodisiac and stimulant (Chopra *et al.* 1956). A decoction of the same is given in flatulent colic and bleeding piles and an infusion is used as eye wash in conjunctivitis. According to Dey (1994), its leaves are chewed to correct foul breath. Chopra *et al.* (1956) told that the seeds are also chewed to correct foul breath and a poultice of the seeds is applied on carbuncles and chronic ulcers. Its watery paste is used as gargle for the cure of mouth and throat ulceration. One pharmaceutical use of coriander is to mask the tastes of other medicinal compounds or to calm the irritating effects on the stomach that some medicines cause.

Coriander has been used as a folk medicine for the relief of anxiety and insomnia in Iranian folk medicine. If used too freely, the seeds become narcotic. All parts of the plant are edible, but the fresh leaves and the dried seeds are the most commonly used in cooking. The leaves have a very different taste from the seeds, similar to parsley but "juicier" and with citrus-like overtones.

Carum Copticum

Vernacular names: Eng: Carom; Hindi: Ajvain; Tam: Omam; German: Adiowan, Ajowan; French: Ajowan

Description: It is the small seed-like fruit, egg-shaped and grayish in colour. The plant has a similarity to parsley. Because of their seed-like appearance, the fruit pods are sometimes called ajwain seeds. Ajwain is annual herbaceous, 30–70 cm (1–2 ft) in height, bearing feathery leaves and red flowers (Fig. 6.5, colour plate 4).

Chemical composition: The major constitutes of the oil of *Carum copticum* are thymol (54.50%), y-terpinene (26.10%) and *p*-cymene (22.10%) (Abdolali *et al.* 2007).

Medicinal uses: The fruits of *C. copticum* have several therapeutic effects including carminative, diuretic and anti-vomiting effects (Abdolali *et al.* 2007).

It is also traditionally known as a digestive aid, relieves abdominal discomfort due to indigestion and as an antiseptic used as a calming herb to ease flatulent dyspepsia and intestinal colic, especially in children. It stimulates the appetite. Its astringency is taken advantage in the treatment of diarrhea, and in laryngitis as a gargle. It is also used in the treatment for bronchitis and bronchial asthma. Several therapeutic effects including anti-asthma and dyspnea have been described for the seeds of *Carum copticum* (Boskabady *et al.* 2005).

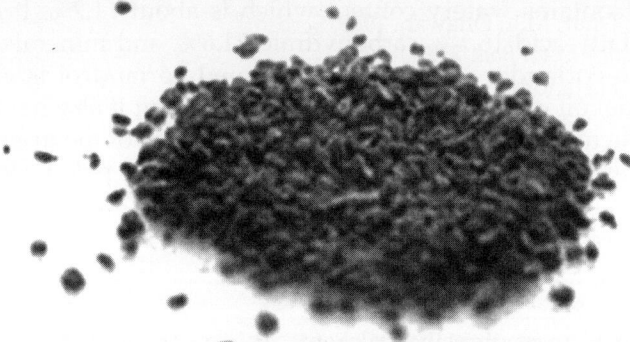

Fig. 6.5: Azwain seeds

It has been used to increase milk flow in nursing mothers. Antispasmodic properties of carum seed can be taken advantage of in soothing the digestive tract, muscles such as uterus, etc. It is also useful for menstrual cramps. *C. copticum* extract possesses a clear-cut analgesic effect (Mohammad *et al*. 2007).

Summary

The present write up covers therapeutic aspects of spice drugs: Cumin, caraway and coriander. These have been used for thousands of centuries by many cultures to enhance the flavor and aroma of foods. Early cultures also recognized the value of using spices and herbs in preserving foods and for their medicinal value. Scientific experiments have documented the antimicrobial properties of some spices, herbs, and their components. In addition to antimicrobial effects, spices and herbs have also shown other disease fighting properties like lowering the cholesterol, stimulating immune system and they are anticancerous and anti-inflammatory also. These work as anti-oxidants and are effective in bronchial asthma. Essential oils extracted from spices and herbs are generally recognized to contain the active antimicrobial compounds. The presence of these compounds, when added to food items, function as inhibitors to the growth of microorganisms in addition to adding flavour and aroma to the food products. Some recent studies regarding the antimicrobial effect of spices and herbs have shown promising results. However, the antimicrobial activity varies widely, depending on the type of spice or herb, test medium, and microorganism. More studies are required in this area to throw further light on the role of spices and herbs as therapeutic agents, particularly keeping in view the increasing reports of resistance of microorganisms to chemotherapeutic agents.

REFERENCES

1. Abdolali M Faridi P, Gasemi Y. 2007. *Carum copticum* Benth. and Hook., essential oil chemotypes. *Food Chemistry*: 10(3): 1217–1219.
2. Ambasta SP. 1986. The useful Plants of India. Publication and Information Directorate CSIR, New Delhi.
3. Aswal BS, Goel AK, Mukherjee KC. 1984. Screening of Indian plants for biological activity (Part-10). *Indian J Expt. Boil*. 22: 321–262.

4. Bhakuni; D.S; Dhar, M.L; Dhawan. 1969, Screening of Indian plants for biological activity (Part- II). *Indian J Expt. Boil.* 7: 250–262.

5. Boskabady M.H., Jandaghi P., Kiani S. and Hasanzadeh L. 2005, Antiussive effect of Carum copticum in guinea pigs. *Journal of Ethnopharmacology*: ,97(1):79–82.

6. Chauhan PS, Satti NK, Suri KA, Amina M, Bani S. 2010, Stimulatory effects of *Cuminum cyminum* and flavanoid glycoside on Cyclosporin- A and ressistant stress induced immuno-suppression in Swiss albino mice. *Chem Bio Intract.* 15;(1): 66–72.

7. Chopra R.N., Nayar S.L. and Chopra I.C., 1956. Glossary of Indian Medicinal Plants. Publications and Information Directorate, C.S.I.R., New Delhi.

8. Dey, A.C. 1994 (Reprint of 1980 Edition). Indian Medicinal Plants used in Ayurvedic Preparations. Bishen Singh Mahendra Pal Singh, Dehradun.

9. Fransworth, N.R., Akerelo, O., Bingel, A.S., Soejarto, D.D. and Guo, Z. 1985, Medicinal plants in therapy. *Bull World Health Organ,* 63:965–981.

10. George A., Burdock, and Ioana G. 2009, Saftey assessment of coriander (*Coriandrum sativum* L.) essential oil as a food ingredient. *Food and Chemical Toxicology.* 47(1), 22–34.

11. Kaushik, P and Dhiman, A.K. 2000, Medicinal Plants and Raw Drugs of India. Bishan Singh Mahendra Pal Singh, Dehradun pp. XII + 1–623.

12. Lacobellis NS, Lo Cantore P, Capasso F, Senalore F. 2005 Jan, Antibacterial activity of *Cuminum cuminum* L. and *Carum carvi* L. essential oil. *J Agric Food Chem:* 12;53(1):57–61.

13. Mohammad HDR, Hajazian S.H., Morshedi A. and Rafati A. 2007, The analgesic effect of *Carum copticum* extract and morphine on phasic pain in mice. *Journal of Ethnopharmacology*: 109 (3), 226–228.

14. Newman, D.J Cragg, G.M. and Snadar, K.M. 2000, The influence of natural products upon drug discovery. *Nat Prod Rep.* 17: 215–234.

15. Patel, V.K, and Bhatt H.V. 1984, *In vitro* antibacterial activity of drug plants. *Indian J. Med. Science.* 2: 34-35.

16. Prescott, L.M; Harley, J.P and Klein, D.A. 2005, Microbiology, 6[th]edition. McGraw Hill, NY, pp XXII + 1–992

17. Samine, A., Obi, C.L., Bessong, P.O. and Namrita L. 2005, Activity profiles of fourteen selected medicinal plants from Rural Venda communities in South Africa against fifteen clinical bacterial species. *African Journal of Biotechnology,* 4(12), 1443–1451.

7

Biotechnological Interventions for Development of New Antimicrobials

Tripti Malik • Padma Singh

The discovery that a mold inhibited growth of *Staphylococcus* by Alexander Fleming (1928) can be considered as an important landmark in the history of medicine. This agent was termed "antibiotic" (Greek *anti*, against, and *bios*, life), defined as microbial products or their derivatives that can kill susceptible microorganisms or inhibit their growth (Prescott et al. 2005). The discovery of antibiotics and their large scale production enabled their widespread use and ushered in the beginning of the "antibiotic era" (Wilcox, 2004). The ' Golden Age' of antibiotic research lasted from the 1940s to the late 1960s, and by the late 1970s, the medical world proclaimed that the battle against infectious agents has been won. Since, antibiotics had a profound effect on human health and contributed to an eight-year increase in the average human lifespan (Hancock and Knowles, 1998). Unfortunately, in early 1990s, humankind has been confronted with an unprecedented number of resurgent and 'new' infectious diseases on a global scale.

Once considered as wonder drugs, the antibiotics are now losing their magical charm as now even the newly introduced antibiotics are becoming ineffective for pathogens. Concurrently, the problem of antibiotic resistance has increased dramatically during the past 10 to 15 years, which poses a serious threat to the treatment of infection. In the last two decades, however, the problem has escalated as the prevalence of antibiotic-resistant bacteria has increased and multi-drug-resistant strains have emerged in many species that cause disease in humans (Conly and Johnston, 2005).

The inappropriate use of antibiotics in the medical environment has also contributed to the problem of antibiotic resistance. A major concern is the use of antibiotics as feed additives given to farm animals to promote animal growth and to prevent infections. This usage contributes to the emergence of antibiotic resistant pathogens and also reduces the effectiveness of an antibiotic to combat human infections. The nontherapeutic use of antibiotics in livestock production accounts for 60% of total antibiotic production in US (Todar, 2008).

Despite the increase in antimicrobial resistance, the development of new antimicrobial agents is declining (Conly and Johnston, 2005). The research and development programs of 15 major pharmaceutical companies and seven major biotechnology companies were examined and it was revealed that FDA approval of new antibacterial agents had decreased by 56% over the past 20 years. Only seven (3%) antibacterial agents have been approved out of total 225 entities by FDA from January 1998 to December 2002 (Spellberg et al. 2004). Conventionally, antimicrobial drugs were developed on the basis of their ability to inhibit bacterial multiplication. However, in the present scenario of antimicrobial resistance, an urgent attention of scientific community is required so that new drug targets should be determined and alternative novel strategies should be explored in order to curb the global menace of antibiotic resistance.

Phytochemicals and Aromachemicals

Medicinal plants have been used as remedies for treatment of human diseases because they contain components of therapeutic value (Nostro et al. 2000). Till so far, more than 30% of the entire plant species have been used for medicinal purposes. Chinese, Indian, Arabian and other traditional systems of medicines make extensive use of about 5000 plants (Thomas, 2000). According to WHO, 80% of the world's population relies on traditional medicine for their healthcare needs (Pierangeli et al. 2009).

In vivo studies have also been done for the antimicrobial assesssment of herbal products. The effect of 'oolong' tea polyphenols on dental caries has been studied in mice (Sakanaka et al., 1992) and on cholera in mice (Toda et al. 1992). The effect of 'ginseng' has been studied in a bacterial infection model, *P. aeruginosa* lung infection of athymic rats. Treated rats had decreased lung pathology and bacterial load, although enhanced humoral immunity was thought to be at least partially responsible (Song et al. 1997). An extract of *Solanum nigrescens*, was given as intravaginal suppositories, in women with confirmed *C. albicans vaginitis*. The extract proved to be as efficacious as the antifungal, nystatin (Giron et al. 1988). Two proprietary compounds derived from tropical plants, Provir, for the treatment of respiratory viral infections, and Virend, a topical antiherpes agent, were tested in clinical trials in 1994 (King et al. 1994). Since then, the efficacy and safety of Virend have been established in phase II studies (Orozco-Topete et al. 1997).

The essence component of plants constitute "quinta-essenia" or essential oil fraction (Lee et al. 2004). Aromachemicals present in different parts of aromatic plants have been widely used in aromatherapy since millennia indicating their therapeutic potential (Thomas, 2000). High antimicrobial activity of essential oils has been determined against food spoilage bacteria and fungi (Aureli et al. 1992; Lis-Balchin et al. 1998; Mangena and Muyima, 1999; Suhr and Neilson, 2003). Hence, essential oils can be the suitable alternative for synthetic preservatives owing to their flavouring, antioxidant and antimicrobial potential. Essential oils such as *Ocimum basilicum*, *Cymbopogon winterianus* and *Mentha arvensis* also show inhibitory activity against pathogens associated with respiratory tract infections (Pant et al. 2008). Essential oils can also be applied for the topical treatment of dermatophytic and candidal infections due to their antifungal properties (Patra et al. 2002; Inouye et al. 2006).

Incorporation of essential oils of *Ocimum basilicum* and *O. gratissimium* in tooth pastes and mouth washes has shown antimicrobial activities against aerobic dental isolates (Akonkahi et al. 2009). Antimicrobial potential of five essential oils namely, basil, chamomile, geranium, lemongrass and thuja against uropathogens has been determined. Geranium oil exhibited best inhibitory activity against both antibiotic sensitive and resistant urinary isolates (Malik and Singh, 2010). Inhibitory activities of essential oils and their components have been determined against different bacterial and fungal isolates.

Probiotics

Probiotics commonly called good bugs, are live microorganisms which when consumed in adequate amounts confer a health benefit on the host (Stealor and Hill, 2008). Several health benefits have been attributed to the ingestion of probiotic bacteria such as *Lactobacillus* sp. and *Bifidobacterium* sp. Probiotic food products have also been called nutraceuticals, pharma foods, designer foods, nutritional foods, medical foods or super foods (Puniya et al. 2008). These bacteria enhance the population of beneficial bacteria in the human gut, suppress pathogens and build up resistance against intestinal diseases. Clinical studies have shown a myriad of impressive health promoting effects of probiotics which includes effective treatment of certain digestive and metabolic disorders (Stealor and Hill, 2008). Antibacterial activity of *Lactobacillus casei* (commercial Yakult drink) against four diarrheagenic microrganisms — ETEC, *Salmonella enteridis*, *Shigella dysentriae* and *Vibrio cholerae* was shown even at 5 minutes effective time (Consignado et al. 1993). Certain probiotic microorganisms have been shown to produce potent antimicrobial peptides (bacteriocins) which specifically target the invading pathogen. For example, nisin and other structurally related lantibiotics use the cell wall precursor lipid II bound to the membrane as a docking molecule for pore formation and inhibition of cell wall biosynthesis. Significant potential of anti-*C. difficile*, a bacteriocin has been proved. The two-component lantibiotic lacticin 3147 completely eliminates 10^6 cfu *C. difficile* ml^{-1}within 30 min without dramatically impacting on the normal resident microflora (Rea et al. 2007). These multiple modes of action significantly reduce the risk of resistance development; hence these can be effectively utilized as an alternative therapeutic agent (Sang and Blecha, 2008). Probiotic products based on this approach have also been formulated against *Clostridium difficile*. However, the physiological instability of probiotic bacteria is a significant limitation for their use in various formulations. The physiological robustness and stress tolerance of probiotic strains can be improved by patho-biotechnology. This novel approach involves the generation of "improved" probiotic strains, using the stress survival systems mined from more physiologically robust pathogenic microbes (Sleator and Hill, 2009). Recently, a single bile resistance gene from the food-borne pathogen *Listeria monocytogenes* has been cloned and expressed in *Bifidiobacterium breve*. This designer probiotic not only had improved gastrointestinal colonization and persistence, but clinical efficacy of probiotic strain was also improved. In an alternative therapeutic preparation, genes for bacteriocin production are introduced into an appropriate bacterial carrier, such as *Lactobacillus salivarius*. This approach circumvents in vivo degradation of the bacteriocin during gastric transit and facilitates continued bacteriocin production in the sigmoid colon, at the same time improving the clinical efficacy of the probiotic. In another approach, designer probiotics have been engineered to express receptor-mimic structures on their surface. When administered orally, these probiotics bind to and neutralize toxins in the gut lumen and interfere with pathogen adherence to the intestinal epithelium, thus mop up the pathogens. Designer probiotics with receptor blocking potential against enterotoxigenic *E. coli* toxin LT and cholera toxin (Ctx) have also been prepared (Paton et al. 2006). In addition to the enteric pathogens, designer probiotics can be used against AIDS. These probiotics express HIV receptors for the virus, which will compete with host cell recptors for the virus, thus providing a natural innate barrier to HIV attachment and infection (Liu et al. 2007).

Designer probiotics can also be used as novel delivery vehicles, which can stimulate both innate and acquired immunities without causing the toxicity reactions (Amdekar et al., 2010). It has been reported at the US biotechnology Industry Organisation 2006 meeting that mother's milk contains a molecule which is 100 times more effective than the most potent form of penicillin, which can be commercially utilised. This molecule is named AGG01, is capable of killing four types of Gram-positive bacteria, and a fungus (Irani, 2006).

Defensins

Natural anti-infective molecules such as antimicrobial peptides constitute a promising strategy for development of new antimicrobials. Approximately 25 years ago, it was discovered that the skin of frogs, the lymph of insects and human neutrophils contain cationic peptides. Till date, 600 cationic peptides have been virtually discovered in virtually all organisms from microbe to man (Wilcox, 2004). These peptides are an important component of the innate defenses to all species of life hence are also known as defensins (Hancock and Lehrer, 1998). Human defensins also play an important role as immune modulators in adaptive immunity (Territo et al. 1989; Yang et al. 1999; Yang et al. 2001). Defensins are cationic, cysteine-rich peptides with molecular masses ranging from 3 to 5 kDa that form characteristic intramolecular disulphide bonds (Selsted and Ouellette, 2005; Leeuw and Lu, 2007). The anti-infective properties of defensins have been well described for a number of viruses (Ref 48 Koltman frm Leeuw and Lu, 2007). The inhibition of HIV has been described by rodent α-defensins (Nakashima et al. 1993), human α-defensins and β-defensins (Wang et al. 2004; Wu et al. 2005).

An insect-derived class of antimicrobial agents known as pyrrhocoricins has been discovered at Philadelphia's Wistar Institute, are active against a range of resistant bacteria. Pyrrhocoricins bind to DnaK, a heat shock protein used to repair faulty bacterial proteins. Inhibition of DnaK causes improper protein synthesis eventually kills the bacterium (Najafi, 2009).

Recombinant DNA procedures are followed for production of small antimicrobial cationic peptides. Bacterial expression systems were employed; a number of different fusion protein systems were tested, including fusions to glutathione-S-transferase (GST) (on plasmid pGEX-KP), *Pseudomonas aeruginosa* outer membrane protein OprF (on plasmid pRW5), *Staphylococcus aureus* protein A (on plasmid pRIT5) and the duplicated IgG-binding domains of protein A (on plasmid pEZZ18). In the first three cases, stable fusion proteins with the defensin, human neurophil peptide 1 (HNP-1), and/or a synthetic cecropin/melittin hybrid (CEME) were obtained. A novel method for purifying inclusion bodies, using the detergent octyl-polyoxyethylene (octyl-POE). Cationic proteins were successfully released from the carrier protein with high efficiency by chemical means (CNBr clevage) and with low efficiency by enzymatic cleavage (using factor Xa protease) (Piers et al. 1993).

Since defensins have antibacterial, antiendotoxic, antibiotic-potentiating or antifungal properties, hence they can be utilized for use as a novel class of antimicrobial agents and for developing disease-resistant plants and animals (Hancock and Lehrer, 1998).

Aganocides and Marine Natural Products

Recently, a novel class of antimicrobial compounds known as aganocides (N, N-dichloro-2, 2-dimethyltaurines) have been described which are effective against MRSA and mupirocin-resistant *Staphyococcus*. Aganocides belong to a class of naturally occurring antimicrobial agents, the N-chlorotaurins that operates within the human immune system and do not give rise to bacterial resistance. Chloronium ions generated by aganocides rapidly inactivate organisms by attacking sulphur- and nitrogen-containing amino acids on the bacterium's surface (Najafi, 2009).

Marine sponges and their associated microorganisms are responsible for more than 5,300 different products, and every year hundreds of new substances are discovered (Faulkner, 2001: 2002). Many marine natural products have successfully advanced to the late stages of clinical trials, e.g. ara-A (vidarabine), an anti-viral drug used against herpes simplex encephalitis virus (De clerq, 2002). Psammaplin A, isolated from the sponge Psammaplysilla, is in preclinical assessment and is the first antibacterial substance to give origin to commercial medication manzamine A (activity against malaria, tuberculosis and HIV) and lasonolides (antifungal activity) derived from marine sponges have also been selected for extended preclinical assessment (Laport et al. 2009).

Lantibiotics

Lantibiotics are gene-encoded peptides that contain the thioether amino acids lanthionine (Lan) and/or methyllanthionine (MeLan) which are formed by post-translational modification and introduce intramolecular cyclic structures. Till so far, 60 lantibiotics have been described. All of these substances are produced by Gram-positive bacteria and they exert their inhibitory action on other Gram-positive bacteria (Bierbaum and Sahl, 2009). They act mainly against Gram-positive bacteria, including some nosocomial pathogens as methicillin resistant *Staphylococcus aureus* (MRSA), enterococci and *Clostridium difficile*. Only some Gram-negative bacteria such as *Moraxella catarrhalis*, *Neisseria gonorrhoeae* and *N. meningitidis* are inhibited by nisin and microbisporicin (Castiglione, 2007).

Nisin was the first lantibiotic to be discovered and was isolated from *Lactococcus lactis*. It is the most prominent among lantibiotics and is employed as a food preservative (Rogers and Whittier, 1928). Nisin shows the strongest antimicrobial activity against multiresistant clinical isolates observed so far for lantibiotics and contains two new post-translational modifications, 5-chloro-tryptophan and bis-hydroxylated proline. Among lantibiotics, nisin shows the strongest antibacterial activity against multiresistant clinical isolates (Castiglione, 2008). The second lantibiotic to be described was subtilin (Jansen and Hirschmann, 1944). Lantibiotics are classified into type A and type B; type A lantibiotics have an elongated flexible configuration and type B lantibiotics are globular peptides. Type A lantibiotics act by binding to lipid II and disturbing the membrane, whereas type-B act by inhibition of enzymes (Jung, 1991). Nisin is also the first lantibiotic to be clinically tested; it has been evaluated as an alternative to intramammary antibiotic for treatment of bovine mastitis in 1940s. The promising results were achieved because of its ability to inhibit a wide range of mastitis causing microorganisms (Taylor, 1949). It has been used successfully in combination with lysostaphin, resulting in cure of 66%, 95% and 100% animals infected with *Staphylococcus aureus, Streptococcus aglactiae* and *Streptococcus uberis* (Sears et al. 1995). Nisin has also been suggested for treatment of superficial skin infections and gastric ulcers. Its sporicidal and antibacterial property is suitable for its application in *Clostridium difficile*-associated diarrhea (Boakes and Wadman, 2008). Lacticin 3147 which is active at physiological pH, has also produced promising results, when incorporated in a teat seal product, an oil-based formulation that forms a physical barrier against infection in the area of teat canal and sinus (Ryan, 1998). Gallidermin and other lantibiotics can be incorporated into the prosthetic joint cement and are being evaluated as prophylactics against implant associated infections. Preliminary tests have been demonstrated that both gallidermin and epidermin are active against *Propionibacterium acnes* (Hancock and Sahl, 2006).

Lantibiotics are ribosomally synthesized peptides. Their structural *lanA* genes are encoded in biosynthetic gene clusters that contain all the genes which are necessary for the introduction of rare amino acids, export, regulation and producer self-protection. The prepeptide consists of an N-terminal leader sequence of up to 59 amino acids in length (cinA) and the C-terminal propeptide part that is modified to be the mature lantibiotic. The modification is performed either by one enzyme, LanM or alternatively a combination of two enzymes, LanB (dehydratase) and LanC(cyclase) that introduces the thioethers (Bierbaum and Sahl, 2009). Several attempts to express and purify the modification enzymes of type-AI lantibiotics have been carried out (Kupke, 1996; Peschel, 1996). The protein engineering studies are being carried on lantibiotics to improve their biological properties and extent of their applications (Cotter et al. 2005). Research has been going on for the construction of lantibiotics with enhanced antimicrobial activity and improved physical properties (solubility, pH stability, heat and protease resistance). For better production of lantibiotic, different biotechnological approaches can be followed which include expression of modified *lanA* genes into the original host, replacement of original *lanA* gene or complementation of an inactivated copy of *lanA* gene in *trans*. Such approaches have been followed for several lantibiotics, e.g. nisin, subtilin, Pep5, epidermin and gallidermin, mutacin II, lacticin 481 and mersacidin (Liu, 1992; Chen, 1998; Szekat, 2003). The whole gene cluster of nisin was sub-cloned and transferred into *Bacillus subtilis* 168 (Yuksel and Hansen, 2007). A plasmid copy harbouring the engineered *mrsA* gene was installed in a σ^H knockout variant of the host.

Apart from modifying lantibiotics, the lantibiotic enzymes may also be applied to biotechnological engineering of other peptides. The thioether rings of lantibiotics convey protection against proteases and other peptides since many biologically active peptides are prone to proteolytic degradation. The introduction of thioether rings will increase half-life, therefore, lower doses, lower administration frequencies and other administration routes become possible (Lubelski, 2008). Lantibiotics can be commercial exploited using relevant fermentation processes. However, the over-production of lantibiotics is hampered by the self-toxicity of the product. Lantibiotics are activated by the cleavage of the leader peptide. Inactivation of the activating protease GdmP led to higher titres of pregallidermin in fed batch fermentations than reached with gallidermin (Valsesia et al. 2007). A promising feature of this class of compounds is their favourable resistance profiles against Gram-positive pathogens and thus current development is likely to focus on the use of lantibiotics as antibacterials (Boakes and Wadman, 2008).

Bacteriophage Therapy

Bacteriophages or phages are bacterial viruses that invade bacterial cells and, in the case of lytic phages, disrupt bacterial metabolism and cause the bacterium to lyse (Abhilash et al. 2009).

Edward Twort (1915) and Felix d'Herelle independently described filterable entities which are called'bacteriophages'. Between 1917 and 1956, some 800 publications dealt with a range of medical applications of bacteriophages. Research was carried in different countries on phage therapy for treatment of different bacterial diseases. However, with the advent of new chemical antibiotics like penicillin, which became widely available in the 1940s, research on the potent but unpredictable phage therapy was abandoned in the western world. During the second advent (in 1980s) of phage therapy, companies in the USA pursued their own approaches towards testified phage therapies, but are still going through trials with their products. In 1997, a patent was issued to the company both for a process of purifying phages that can circulate for a long time in the blood, and for their use to treat infections in animals and humans (Lorch, 1999). During the long history of their usuage as therapeutic agents in Eastern Europe and Soviet Union, phages have been administered humans by different routes, viz. orally, rectally, locally, intravenously, as aerosols, there have been no reported serious complications (Sulakvelidze, 2001). Despite the *in vitro* clinical efficacy of bacteriophages, the approval for commercial preparations of phages has not been permitted. Indeed some phage companies are planning towards the commercialisation of phage products for agricultural applications, where regulations are less stringent (Thiel, 2004).

Working with the filamentous coliphage M13, the researchers created a sort of zombie phage — a regular phage body that still seeks out a specific microbial host (in this case, *E. coli*) but that has had its head emptied of the usual DNA necessary for replication. It instead injects only a lethal protein system, killing the host cell but not leading to the lysis of the cell or new phage production (Thiel, 2004). A newer concept is of enzybiotics, which are the phage-coded lysins that destroy the cell wall of bacteria. A rapid killing of *Streptococcus pneumoniae* in the nasopharynx of mice has been described using a phage-coded murein hydrolase in a murine sepsis model. Hence, the therapy with enzybiotics against pneumococcus constitutes an alternative strategy for treatment of diseases causing bacteremia and death (Jado et al. 2003).

A matter of concern regarding their therapeutic application is that, phages that are directly lethal to bacterial host cells may lead to selection of phage resistant bacteria in short time (Summers, 2001). Engineered bacteriophage can offer a solution; bacteriophages have been engineered to overexpress proteins and attack gene networks that are not directly targeted by antibiotics. Engineered phages have been designed by suppressing the SOS network in *E. coli*, which enhances killing by quinolones by several orders of magnitude *in vitro* and hence increases the survival of infected mice *in vivo* (Lu and Collins, 2008).

Antisense Therapy

Antisense agents have received widespread interest as potential therapeutic agents for a number of diseases, including cancer, inflammatory conditions and viral infections. It is also evident that antisense agents can be specifically targeted to genes that control expression of antibiotic resistance mechanisms, thereby potentially restoring an antibiotic-sensitive phenotype to the cell (Chopra, 1999). The 'antisense' or 'antigene' agents are used to inhibit resistance mechanisms at the nucleic acid level. Strictly, 'antisense' and 'antigene' (hereafter referred to collectively as antisense) oligonucleotides bind mRNA to prevent translation or bind DNA to prevent gene transcription, respectively. Interrupting expression of resistance genes in this manner could restore susceptibility to key antibiotics, which would be co-administered with the antisense compound (Woodford and Warehem, 2009).

Peptide nucleic acids (PNAs) attached to short carrier peptides can be used as antisense agents to downregulate the expression of specific proteins in *Staphylococcus aureus*. PNA is an uncharged and stable DNA mimic. In order to facilitate the entry of PNAs into the bacteria across the cell wall, these are attached to cationic carrier peptides (Nekhotiaeva et al., 2004). Previously, PNA-antisense antibiotics have been directed towards the start codon region of specific genes were applied for down regulation in *E. coli* (Good and Nielsen, 1998).

Antisense therapy may have a role in prevention of dental plaque, which is caused due to biofilm of *Streptococcus mutans* adherent cells separated by fluid-filled spaces in a capsular polysaccharide matrix. Anti-gtfB antrisense PS-oligonucleotides inhibit gtfB transcription, expression and the biofilm formation by *S. mutans*. It can be used as a novel reagent against *S. mutans cariogenesis* (Guo et al. 2006).

REFERENCES

1. Abhilash M, Vidya AG, Jagadevi T. 2009. Bacteriophage therapy: A war against antibiotic resistant bacteria. *The Internet Journal of Alternative Medicine* 7 (1).
2. Akonkahi I, Ayinde BA, Edogun O, Uhuwmangho MU. 2009. Antimicrobial activities of the volatile oils of Ocimum bacilicum and Ocimum gratissimum L. (Lamiaceae) against some aerobic dental isolates. *Pak. J. Pharm. Sci.* 22: 405–409.
3. Amdekar S, Dwivedi D, Roy P. et al. 2010. Probiotics: multifarious oral vaccine against infectious traumas. *FEMS Immunol Med Microbiol.* 58: 299–306.
4. Aureli, P., Costantini, A. and Zolea, S. 1992. Antimicrobial activity of some plant essential oils against Listeria monocytogenes. *Journal of Food Protection* 55, 344–348.
5. Bierhaum, G. and Sahl, H.G. 2009. Lantibiotics: mode of action, biosynthesis and bioengineering. *Current Pharmaceutrical Biotechnology.* 10: 2–18.
6. Boakes, S. and Wadman, S. 2008. The therapeutic potential of lantibiotics. *Drug Discovery and Development* 27:22–25.

7. Castiglione, F., Cavaletti, L., Losi, D., Lazzarini, A., Carrano. L., Feroggio, M., Ciciliato, I., Corti, E., Marinelli, F. and Selva, E. 2007. Important classes of antibiotics acting on bacterial cell wall biosynthesis. *Biochemistry* 46 (20): 5884–5895.

8. Castiglione, F., Lazzarini, A., Carrano, L., Corti, E., Ciciliato, I., Gastaldo, L., Candiani, P., Losi, D., Marinelli, F., Selva, E. and Parenti, F. 2008. Determining the structure and mode of action of microbisporicin, a potent lantibiotic active against multiresistant pathogens. *Chem. Biol.* 15 (1): 22–31.

9. Chen, P., Novak, J., Kirk, M., Barnes, S., Qi, F. and Caufield, P.W. 1998. Structure-activity study of the lantibiotic mutacin II from Streptococcus mutans T8 by a gene replacement strategy. *Appl. Environ. Microbiol.* 64 (7): 2335–2340s.

10. Chopra, I. 1999. *Prospects for Antisense Agents in the Therapy of Bacterial Infections.* 8(8): 1203–1208.

11. Conly, J.M. and Johnston, B.L. 2005. Where are all the new antibiotics? The new antibiotic paradox. *Can J Infect Dis Med Microbiol.* 16 (3): 159–160.

12. Consignado, G.O., Pena, A.C. and Jacalne, A. 1993. In vitro study on the antibacterial activity of *Lactobacillus casei* (commercial yakult drink) against four diarrhea-causing organisms. *Phil J Microbiol Infect Dis.* 22 (2): 50–55.

13. Cotter, P.D., Hill, C. and Ross, R.P. 2005. Bacterial lantibiotics: strategies to improve therapeutic potential. *Current Protein and Peptide Science* 6:61–75.

14. De Clerq, E. 2002. New anti-HIV agents and targets. *Med. Res. Rev.* 22: 531–565.

15. Faulkner, D.J. 2001. Marine natural products. *Nat. Prod. Rep.* 19: 1–48.

16. Faulkner, D.J. 2002. Marine natural products. *Nat. Prod. Rep.* 18: 1–49.

17. Giron, L. M., Aguilar, G. A., Caceres, A. and Arroyo, G. L. 1988. Anticandidal activity of plants used for the treatment of vaginitis in Guatemala and clinical trial of a Solanum nigrescens preparation. *J. Ethnopharmacol.* 22: 307–313.

18. Good, L., and Nielsen, P.E. 1998. Antisense inhibition of gene expression in bacteria by PNA targeted to mRNA. *Nature Biotechnology* 16: 355–358.

19. Guo Q-Y., Xiao, G., Li, R., Guan S., Zhu, X. and Wu, J. 2006. Treatment of Streptococcus mutans with antisense oligodeoxyribonucleotides to gtfB mRNA inhibits GtfB expression and function. *FEMS Microbiol Lett.* 264: 8–14.

20. Hancock R.E. and Lehrer, R. 1998. Cationic peptides: a new source of antibiotics. *Trends Biotechnology.* 16 (2): 82–88.

21. Hancock, R. and Knowles, D. 1998. Are we approaching the end of the antibiotic era? *Current Opinion in Microbiology* 1:493–494.

22. Hancock, R.E.W. and Sahl, H.G. 2006. Antimicrobial and host defense peptides as new anti infection therapeutic strategies. *Nature Biotechnology* 24 (12): 551–557.

23. Inouye, S., Uchida, K. and Abe, S. 2006. Vapour activity of 72 essential oils against a Trichophyton mentagrophytes. *Journal of Infection and Chemotherapy* 12 (4), 210–216.

24. Irani, 2006. Milk to fight against antibiotics 100 times more effectively than penicillin. http://www.ecofriend.org.

25. Jado, I., Lopez R., Garcia, E., Fenoll, A., Casal, J. and Garcia P. 2003. Phage lytic enzymes as therapy for antibiotic-resistant Streptococcus pneumoniae infection in a murine sepsis model. *Journal of Antimicrobial Chemotherapy* 52: 967–973.

26. Jansen, E.F. and Hirschmann, D.J. 1944. Subtilin, an antibacterial product of Bacillus subtilis: culturing conditions and properties. *Arch. Biochem.* 4: 297–304.

27. Jung, G. 1991. Nisin and novel lantibiotics. Angew. Chem. Int. Ed. Engl. 30: 1051-1068.

28. King, S. R., and Tempesta, M. S. 1994. From shaman to human clinical trials: the role of industry in ethnobotany, conservation and community reciprocity. *Ciba Found. Symp.* 185: 197–206.

29. Kupke, T. and Gotz, F. 1996. Expression, purification and characterization of epic, an enzyme involved in the biosynthesis of the lantibiotic epidermin, and sequence analysis of Staphylococcus epidermidis epic mutants. *J. Bacteriol.* 178 (5): 1335–1340.

30. Laport, M.S., Santos, O.C.S. and Muricy, G. 2009. Marine sponges: potential sources of new antimicrobial drugs. *Current Pharmaceutical Biotechnology* 10: 86–105. E. J.

31. Lee, K.W., Everts, H. and Benyen, A.C. 2004. Essential oils in broiler nutrition. *International J of Poultry Science* 3 (12): 738–752.

32. Leeuwx, E de and Lu, W. Human defensins: turning defense into offense? 2007. *Infectious Disorders-Drug Targets.* 7: 67–70.

33. Lis-Balchin, M., Buchbauer, G., Hirtenlehner, T. and Resch, M. 1998. Antimicrobial activity of Pelargonium essential oils added to a quiche filling as a model food system. *Letters in Applied Microbiology* 27 (4), 207–210.

34. Liu, J.J., Jiang, Y., Turner, M.S. and Tsai, C.C. 2007. Activity of HIV entry and fusion inhibitors expressed by the human vaginal colonizing probiotic *Lactobacillus reuteri. Cell. Microbiol.* 9: 120–130.

35. Liu, W. and Hansen, J.N. 1992. Enhancement of the chemical and antimicrobial properties of subtilin by site-directed mutagenesis. *J. Biol. Chem.* 267 (35) : 25078–25085.

36. Lorch, A. 1999. "Bacteriophages: An alternative to antibiotics?" *Biotechnology and Development Monitor* 39.pp. 14–17.

37. Lu, T.K. and Collins, J.J. 2009. Engineered bacteriophage targeting gene networks as adjuvants for antibiotic therapy. *PNAS.* 106 (12): 4629–4634.

38. Lubelski, J., Rink, R., Khusainov, R., Moll, G.N. and Kuipers, O.P. 2008 Biosynthesis, immunity, regulation, mode of action and engineering of the model lantibiotic nisin. *Cell Mol. Life Sci.* 65 (3): 455–476.

39. Malik, T. and Singh, P. 2010. Antimicrbial effects of essential oils against uropathogens with varying sensitivity to antibiotics. *Asian Journal of Biological Sciences.* 3 (2): 92–98.

40. Mangena, T. and Muyima, N.Y.O. 1999. Comparative evaluation of the antimicrobial activities of essential oils of Artemisia afra, Pteronia incana and Rosamarinus officinalis on selected bacteria and yeast strains. *Letters in Applied Microbiology* 28 (4), 291–296.

41. Najafi, R. 2009. *Case Study: Overcoming Antimicrobial Resistance.* 29 (4): 1–4.

42. Nekhotiaeva, N., Kumar, S., Awasthi, Nielsen, P.E. and Good, L. 2004. Inhibition of Staphylococcus aureus gene expression and growth using anti-sense therapy. *Molecular Therapy.* 10, 652–659.

43. Nostro, A., Germano, M., Dangelo, V. and Cannatelli, M. 2000. Extraction methods for evaluation of medicinal plant antimicrobial activity. *Lett. Appl. Microbiol.* 30: 379–384.

44. Orozco-Topete, R., Sierra-Madero, J., Cano-Dominguez, C., Kershenovich, J., Ortiz-Pedroza, G., Vazquez-Valls, E., Garcia-Cosio, C., Soria-Cordoba, A., Armendariz, A. M., Teran-Toledo, X., Romo-Garcia, J., Fernandez, H., and Rozhon, E. J. 1997. Safety and efficacy of Virend for topical treatment of genital and anal herpes simplex lesions in patients with AIDS. *Antiviral Res.* 35: 91–103.

45. Pant, S., Malik, T., Deep, B., Chauhan, N. and Lohani, H. 2008. Antimicrobial activity of essential oils on isolates responsible for upper respiratory tracty infection (URTI). *Journal of Medicinal and Aromatic Plant Sciences* 30, 310–313.

46. Paton, A.W., Morona, R. and Paton, J.C. 2010. Receptor-mimic probiotics: potential therapeuticsb for bacterial toxin-mediated enteric diseases. *Expert. Rev. Gastroenterol. Hepatol.* 4: 253–255.

47. Patra, M., Shahi, S.K., Midgely, G. and Dikshit, A. 2002. Utilization of essential oil as natural antifungal against nail-infective fungi. *Flavour and Fragrance Journal* 17, 91–94.

48. Peschel, A., Ottenwalder, B. and Gotz, F. 1996. Inducible production and cellular location of the epidermin biosynthetic enzyme EpiB using an improved staphylococcal expression system. *FEMS Microbiol Lett.* 137 (2–3): 279–284.

49. Pierangeli, G., Vial, G. and Rivera, L. W. 2009. Antimicrobial activity and cytotoxicity of Chromoloena odorata (L. f) King and Robinson and Uncaria perrotietii (A. Rich). Merr. Extracts. *Journal of Medicinal Plants Research* 3 (7); 511–518.

50. Piers, K.L., Brown, M.H. and Hancock, R.E. 1993. Recombinant DNA procedures for producing small antimicrobial cationic peptides in bacteria. *Gene* 134 (1): 7–13.

51. Prescott, L.M., Harley, J.P. and Klein, C.A. Antimicrobial chemotherapy. In: *Microbiology*. 6th edition. McGraw Hill, Singapore. pp. 779–798.

52. Puniya, A.K., Puniya, M., Nagpal, R., Malik, M., Kumar, S., Mishra, V., Dhewa, T., Pant, S. and Singh, K. 2008. Functional dairy foods: a healthy hope. In: Lecture notes: workshop on biotechnology education, Kumar, A., Sahal, G. and Kaur, R.P.(Eds.). pp. 197–205.

53. Rea, M.C., Clayton, E., O'Connor, P.M., Shahahan, F., Kiely, B., Ross, R.P. and Hill, C. 2007. Antimicrobial activity of lacticin 3147 against clinical Clostridium difficle strains. *J Med Microbiol.* 56: 940–946.

54. Rogers, L.A. and Whittier, E.O. 1928. Limiting factors in the lactic fermentation. *J Bacteriol.* 16: 211–229.

55. Ryan, M.P., Meaney, W.J., Ross, R.P. and Hill, C. 1998. Evaluation of lacticin 3147 and a teat seal containing this bacteriocin for inhibition of mastitis pathogens. *Appl. Environ. Microbiol.* 64: 2287–2290.

56. Sakanaka, S., Shimura, N., Aizawa, M., Kim, M. and Yamamoto, T. 1992. Preventive effect of green tea polyphenols against dental caries in conventional rats. *Biosci. Biotechnol. Biochem.* 56: 592–594.

57. Sang, Y. and Blecha, F. 2008. Antimicrobial peptides and bacteriocins: alternatives to trditional antibiotics. *Anim. Health Res. Rev.* 9: 227–235.

58. Sears, P., Peele, J., Lassauzet, M. and Blackburn, P. 1995. Use of antimicrobial proteins in the treatment of bovine mastitis. pp. 17-18. In Proceedings of the 3rd International Mastitis Seminar, TelAviv, Isarel.

59. Selsted, M.E. and Ouellette, A.J. 2005. Mammalian defensins in the antimicrobial immune response. *Nat Immunology.* 6: 551.

60. Song, Z. J., Johansen, H. K., Faber, V. and Hoiby, N. 1997. Ginseng treatment enhances bacterial clearance and decreases lung pathology in athymic rats with chronic Pseudomonas aeruginosa pneumonia. *APMIS* 105: 438–444.

61. Spellberg, B., Powers, J.H., Brass, E.P., Miller, L.G. and Edwards, J.E. 2004. Trends in antimicrobial drug development: Implications for the future. Clin Infect Dis.38: 1279–1286.

62. Stealor, H. and Hill, C. 2008. Designer probiotics: a potential therapeutic for *Clostridium difficile*. *Journal of Medical Microbiology.* 57: 793–794.

63. Stealor, R.D. and Hill, C. 2009. Rational design of improved pharmabiotics. *J Biomed Biotechnology.* 87: 2752.

64. Suhr, K. I. and Nielsen, P.V. 2003. Antifungal activity of essential oils evaluated by two different techniques against rye bread spoilage fungi. *Journal of Applied Microbiology* 94 (4), 665–674.

65. Sulakvelidze, A., Alavidze, Z. and Morris, J.G. 2001. Bacteriophage therapy. *Antimicrobial Agents and Chemotherapy.* 45 (3): 649–659.

66. Summers, W.C. 2001. Bacteriophage therapy. *Annu. Rev. Microbiol.* 55: 437–451. Lu, T.K. and Collins, J.J. 2009. Engineered bacteriophage targeting gene networks. *PNAS.* 106 (12): 9631–9634.

67. Szekat, C., Jack, R.W., Skutlarek, D., Farber, H. and Bierbaum, G. 2003. Construction of an Expression System for Site-Directed Mutagenesis of the Lantibiotic Mersacidin. *Appl. Environ. Microbiol.* 69 (7): 3777–3783.

68. Taylor, J.I., Hirsch, A. and Mattick, A.T.R. 1949. The treatment of bovine streptococcal and staphylococcal mastitis with nisin. *Vet. Rec.* 197–198.

69. Territo, M.C., Ganz, T., Selsted, M.E., Lehrer, R. 1989. Monocyte-chemotactic activity of defensins from human neutrophils. *J Clin Invest.* 84: 2017–2020.

70. Thiel, K. 2004. Old dogma, new tricks- 21st century phage therapy. *Nature Biotechnology.* 22: 31–36.

71. Thomas, J., Joy, P. P., Mathew, S. and Skaria, B. P. 2000. Plant sources of aroma chemicals and medicines in India. *Chemical Industry Digest* (Special millennium issue) 104–108.

72. Toda, M., Okubo, S., Ikigai, H., Suzuki, T., Suzuki, Y., Hara, Y. and Shimamura, T. 1992. The protective activity of tea catechins against experimental infection by *Vibrio cholerae* O1. *Microbiol. Immunol.* 36: 999–1001.

73. Todar, K. 2008. Antimicrobial agents in the treatment of infectious disease. In: Todar's online Textbook of Bacteriology. http://www.textbookofbacteriology.net/antimicrobial. html

74. Valsesia, G., Medaglia, G., Held, M., Minas W. and Panke, S. 2007. Circumventing the Effect of Product Toxicity: Development of a Novel Two-Stage Production Process for the Lantibiotic Gallidermin. *Appl Environ. Microbiol.* 73 (5): 1635–1645.

75. Wang, W., Owen, S.M., Rudolph, D.L., Cole, A.M., Hong, T., Waring, A.J., Lal, R.B. and Lehrer, R.I. *J. Immunol* 2004. 173: 515.

76. Wilcox, S. 2004. The new antimicrobials: cationic peptides. *BioTeach Journal* 2: 88–92.

77. Wilcox, S. The new antimicrobials: cationic peptides. *Bioteach Journal* 2: 88–91.

78. Woodford, N., and Wareham, D.W. 2009. Tackling antibiotic resistance: a dose of common antisense? *Journal of Antimicrobial Chemotherapy* 63 (2): 225–229.

79. Wu, Z., Cocchi, F., Gentles, D., Ericksen ,B., Lubkowski, J., Devico, A., Lehrer, R.I. and Lu, W. 2005. Human neutrophil alpha-defensin 4 inhibits HIV-1 infection *in vitro"*. *FEBS Lett.* 579: 162–166.

80. Yang, D., Chertov, O. and Oppenheim, J.J. 2000. The role of mammalian antimicrobial peptides and proteins in awakening of innate host defenses and adaptive immunity. *J Leukoc. Biol.* 68: 9.

81. Yang, D., Chertov, O., Bylovskaia, Chen, S.N., Buffo, M.J., Shogan, J., Anderson, M., Schroder, J.M., Wang, J.M., Howard, O.M. and Oppenheim, J.J. 1999. *Human neutrophil defensins Science* 286: 525–528.

82. Yuksel, S. and Hansen, J.N. 2007. Transfer of nisin gene cluster from Lactococcus lactis ATCC 11454 into the chromosome of Bacillus subtilis 168. *Appl Microbiol. Biotechnol.* 74 (3): 640–649.

8

Production of Biofuels through Termites and Other New Approaches

Gunjan Sood • Yamini Singh Sisodia • Pradeep Parihar

INTRODUCTION

Biofuel is defined as solid, liquid or gaseous fuel obtained from lifeless or living biological material and is similar to fossil fuels, which are derived from long dead biological material. Also, various plants and plant-derived materials are used for biofuel manufacturing. Biofuel has the added advantage of biosequestration of atmospheric CO_2 and so assisting to remediate greenhouse gas and climate change problems (Adler et al., 2007).

Globally, biofuels are most commonly used to power vehicles, heat homes, and for cooking. Biofuel industries are expanding in Europe, Asia, and America. Los Alamos National Lab have taken out research for the conversion of pollution into renewable biofuel.

Agrofuels are biofuels which are produced from specific crops, rather than from waste processes such as landfill off-gassing or recycled vegetable oil. There are two common strategies of producing liquid and gaseous agrofuels. One is to grow crops high in sugar (sugar cane, sugar beet, and sweet sorghum) or starch (corn/maize), and then use yeast fermentation to produce ethyl alcohol (ethanol) (Tokuda et al., 2007). The second is to grow plants that contain high amounts of vegetable oil, such as oil palm, soybean, algae, jatropha, or Pongamia pinnata.

When these oils are heated, their viscosity is reduced, and they can be burned directly in a diesel engine, or they can be chemically processed to produce fuels such as biodiesel. Wood and its byproducts can also be converted into biofuels such as woodgas, methanol or ethanol fuel (Pu et al., 2007). It is also possible to make cellulosic ethanol from non-edible plant parts, but this can be difficult to accomplish economically. Biofuels can be produced in large quantities and have multiple benefits, but only if they come from feedstocks produced with low life cycle greenhouse gas emissions, as well as minimal competition with food production. This consensus emerges in a new journal article by researchers from the University of Minnesota, Princeton, MIT and the University of California, Berkeley (Pu *et al*, 2007).

PRODUCTION OF BIOFUELS

Biofuel is considered to be the most pure and the easiest available fuels on the planet. Also known as agrofuel, they are classified into gas, liquid and solid form derived from biomass. Most of the people would be very happy to know that most of the forms of biofuels can be easily manufactured even at in one's kitchen garden. One of the key features of biofuels is that they are better than other forms of fuels like petrol or diesel that is manufactured by most of the big oil manufacturing companies. Most of the diesel engines would work more efficiently and even last longer with the use of these home made biofuels and are also very clean and environment friendly. These biofuels can be a lot more economic, if used in the kitchen for cooking purpose and also encourage the recycling process as most of them are manufactured from waste products (Farrell *et al.*, 2006).

There are various forms of biofuels and most of them are made through a detailed process having various stages. Most of the animal fats, vegetables and oils contain glycerin and are thus called triglycerides. In the process of manufacturing the biofuels, all the fats and oils are turned into esters, separating the glycerin. At the end of the process, all the glycerin sinks down at the bottom and all the biofuel rests at the top. The process through which the glycerin is separated from the biodiesel is known as transesterification (Hill *et al.*, 2006). This process also uses dye as a catalyst in the whole process. Some of the chemicals which are used in the manufacturing of biofuels are ethanol or methanol which brings into use methyl esters. Methanol is derived from fossil fuels while ethanol is derived from plants. One of the advantages of using ethanol is that they can be distilled even at home without any problem.

The process of manufacturing biofuel can be classified in the following stages:

1. *Filtering:* In this process, waste vegetable oil is filtered to remove all the food particles. This process generally involves warming up the liquid a little. After warming up the liquid, it can be filtered with the use of coffee filter.

2. *Removing of water:* All the water contained in the residual gangue has to be removed which will make the reaction faster. The water can be easily removed by making the liquid boil at 100°C for some time.

3. *Titration:* This process is carried out to determine the amount of lye that would be required. This process is the most crucial and the most important stage of biofuel manufacturing.

4. *Preparation of sodium methoxide:* Now methanol is mixed with sodium hydroxide to produce sodium methoxide. In most of the cases, the quantity of methanol used is generally 20% of waste vegetable oil.

5. *Heating and mixing:* The residue is heated in between 120 to 130°F after which it is mixed well. It should be remembered that process should be done carefully avoiding splashing of the liquid.

6. *Settling and separation:* After mixing the liquid, it has to be allowed to cool down. After the cooling process, the biofuel will be found floating at the top while the

heavier glycerin would be found at the bottom. The glycerin can be easily separated by allowing it to drain out from the bottom. The person is left over with pure biofuel which can be used for various purposes (Farrell *et al.*, 2006).

TYPES OF BIOFUEL

Vegetable oil is used in several old diesel engines that have indirect injection systems. This oil is also used to create biodiesel, which when mixed with conventional diesel fuel is compatible for most diesel engines. Used vegetable oil is converted into biodiesel. Sometimes, water and particulates are separated from the used vegetable oil and then this is used as a fuel (Eggleston *et al.*, 2006).

Biodiesel composition is just like mineral diesel. When biodiesel is mixed with mineral diesel, the mixture can be used in any diesel engine. It is observed that in several nations, the diesel engines under warranty are converted to 100% biodiesel use. It has also been proved that most people can run their vehicles on biodiesel without any problem (Richards *et al.*, 1997).

A large number of vehicle manufacturers recommended the use of 15% biodiesel mixed with mineral diesel. In Europe, 5% biodiesel blend is generally used at gas stations (Adler *et al.*, 2007). Bioalcohols are biologically produced alcohols. Common among these are ethanol and rare among these are propanol and butanol. Biobutanol can be used directly in a gasoline engine and hence is considered a direct replacement for gasoline. The butanol can be burned straight in the existing gasoline engines without any alteration to the engine or car. It is also claimed that this butanol produces more energy. Also, butanol has a less corrosive effect and is less soluble in water than ethanol (Eggleston *et al.*, 2006). Ethanol fuel is the most commonly used biofuel in the world and particularly in Brazil. Ethanol can be put to use in petrol engines as a substitute for gasoline. Also, it can be mixed with gasoline in any ratio. The contemporary automobile petrol engines can work on mixtures of gasoline and ethanol that have 15% bioethanol. This mixture of gasoline and ethanol has more quantity of octane. This indicates that the engine would burn hotter and more efficiently. In high altitude spots, the mixture of gasoline and ethanol is used as a winter oxidizer and thereby atmospheric pollution is decreased (Farrell *et al.*, 2006).

The ethanol fuel has less British Thermal Unit energy content. Thus, to drive the same distance, more fuel is required. Also ethanol has a corrosive effect on combustion chambers, aluminum, rubber hoses gaskets and fuel systems. Biogas is created, when organic material is anaerobically digested by anaerobes. During production, there is a solid byproduct called digestate. This can be used as a biofuel or fertilizer. Biogas consists of methane. Landfill gas is created in landfills due to natural anaerobic digestion and is a less clean form of biogas. Dried manure, charcoal and wood are examples of solid biofuels.

The combined processes of gasification, combustion and pyrolyis give rise to **Syngas** which is a biofuel. This syngas can be directly burned in internal combustion engines. Syngas can be used to create hydrogen and methanol. By using the Fischer-Tropsch process, it can be transformed to a synthetic petroleum substitute.

Some second generation biofuels that are being developed are Fischer-Tropsch diesel, biomethanol, biohydrogen, wood diesel, mixed alcohol and biohydrogen diesel. Algae fuel is a third generation biofuel derived from algae. This is also called as **oilgae** (Pu *et al.*, 2007).

The world is facing a potential energy crisis due to fossil fuel energy demand and population increase. Pollution from fossil fuels affects public health, and causes global climate change because of carbon dioxide (CO_2) release. One of the ideas to solve this problem is to use microorganisms that can provide both renewable energy and CO_2 removal from the atmosphere.

Thermophilic, or **heat-loving**, bacteria inhabit Iceland's hot springs, the scientists "bioprospected" scalding-hot geothermal springs in different parts of the country for new ethanol and hydrogen-producing bacteria. After screening samples, including those from springs that approached the boiling point of water, the scientists enriched promising microorganisms that can produce the compounds from glucose or cellulose at high temperatures. The enrichments included those with unusually high yields of hydrogen or ethanol from carbohydrates. Bioprospectors hav identified hot new biofuel-producing bacteria.

Bioethanol Conventional Production

Bioethanol is the most common biofuel, accounting for more than 90% of total biofuel usage. Conventional production is a well-known process based on enzymatic conversion of starchy biomass into sugars, and fermentation of 6-carbon sugars with final distillation of ethanol to fuel grade. Ethanol can be produced from many feedstocks, including cereal crops, corn (maize), sugar cane, sugar beets, potatoes, sorghum, cassava. Coproducts (e.g. animal feed) help to reduce production cost. If sugar cane is used, conversion into sugar is easier (Lal, 2005).

Crushed stalk (bagasse) can be used to provide heat and power for the process and for other energy applications.

The world's largest producers of bio-ethanol are Brazil (sugar cane ethanol) and United States (corn ethanol). Ethanol is used in low 5–10% blends with gasoline (E5, E10) but also as E-85 in flex-fuel vehicles. In Brazil, gasoline must contain a minimum of 22% bioethanol.

Bioethanol Advanced Production

While conventional processes use only the sugar and starch biomass components, R and D focuses on advanced processes that utilise all available ligno-cellulosic materials. These processes hold the potential to increase variety and quantity of suitable feedstock including cellulosic wastes, maize stover, cereal straw, foodprocessing wastes, as well as dedicated fast-growing plants such as poplar trees and switch-grass. Cellulosic feedstock could be grown on non-arable land or be produced from integrated crops, which could considerably increase land availability.

Ethanol production from ligno-cellulosic feedstock includes biomass pre-treatment to release cellulose and hemicellulose, hydrolysis to release fermentable 5- and 6-carbon sugars, sugar fermentation, separation of solid residues and non-hydrolysed cellulose, and distillation to fuel grade. To provide better conversion, new chemical and enzymatic processes (pre-treatment, hydrolysis, fermentation) are being examined. Solid residues and coproducts from the process such as lignin and other components, particularly from forest materials, may inhibit hydrolysis. They can be extracted and used as a fuel in the production process, thus reducing cost and emissions (Prather *et al.*, 2001).

Biodiesel Production

Biodiesel production is based on trans-esterification of vegetable oils and fats through the addition of methanol (or other alcohols) and a catalyst, giving glycerol as a co-product. Feedstock includes rapeseeds, sunflower seeds, soy seeds and palm oil seeds from which the oil is extracted chemically or mechanically.

Advanced processes include the replacement of methanol of fossil origin, by bioethanol to produce fatty acid ethyl ester instead of fatty acid methyl ether (the latter being the traditional biodiesel). In order to expand the relatively small resource base of biodiesel, new processes have been developed to use recycled cooking oils and animal fats though these are limited in volume.

Hydrogenation of oil and fat is a new process that is entering the market. It can produce a biodiesel that can be blended with fossil diesel up to 50% without any engine modifications. Synthetic biofuel production via biomass gasification and catalytic conversion to liquid using Fischer-Tropsch process (biomass conversion to liquids BTL) offers a variety of potential biofuel production processes that may be suited to current and future engine technologies. The largest biodiesel producer is Germany, which accounts for 50% of global production. Biodiesel is currently most often used in 5–20% blends (B5, B20) with conventional diesel, or even in pure B100 form (Prather *et al.*, 2001).

ENERGY INPUT AND EMISSIONS

Fossil energy inputs and emissions levels from biofuel production are sensitive to process and feedstock, to energy embedded in fertilizers, and to local conditions.

Production of ethanol from sugar cane (Brazil) is energy-efficient since the crop produces high yields per hectare and the sugar is relatively easy to extract. If bagasse is used to provide the heat and power for the process, and ethanol and biodiesel are used for crop production and transport, the fossil energy input needed for each ethanol energy unit can be very low compared with 60–80% for ethanol from grains. As a consequence, ethanol well-towheels CO_2 emissions can be as low as 0.2–0.3 $kgCO_2/$ litre ethanol compared with 2.8 kg $CO_2/$litre for conventional gasoline (90% reduction). Ethanol from sugar beet requires more energy input and provides 50–60% emission reduction compared with gasoline.

Ethanol production from cereals and corn (maize) can be even more energy-intensive and debate exists on the net energy gain. Estimates, which are very sensitive to the process used, suggest that ethanol from maize may displace petroleum use by up to 95%, but total fossil energy input currently amounts to some 60–80% of the energy contained in the final fuel (20% diesel fuel, the rest being coal and natural gas) and hence the CO_2 emissions reduction may be as low as 15–25% vs. gasoline.

Ethanol from Lignocellulosic Feedstock

At present, the total energy input needed for the production process may be even higher as compared to bioethanol from corn, but in some cases most of such energy can be provided by the biomass feedstock itself. Net CO_2 emissions reduction from lignocellulosic ethanol can, therefore, be close to 70% vs. gasoline, and could approach 100% if electricity co-generation displaced gas or coal-fired electricity. It is under process research to exploit the large potential from improving efficiency in enzymatic hydrolysis.

Energy input and overall emissions for **biodiesel** production also depend on feedstock and process. Typical values are fossil fuel inputs of 30% and CO_2 emission reductions of 40–60% vs. diesel. Using recycled oils and animal fats reduces the CO_2 emissions.

ENERGY FROM BIO-WASTE

European Union highlighted the potential for waste-derived bioenergy to contribute to the reduction of global warming. A European report concluded that the equivalent of 19 million tons of oil is available from biomass by 2020, 46% from bio-wastes — municipal solid waste (MSW), agricultural residues, farm waste and other biodegradable waste streams (Marshall *et al.*, 2007).

Landfill sites generate gases as the waste buried in them undergoes anaerobic digestion. These gases are known collectively as landfill gas (LFG). This is considered a source of renewable energy, even though landfill disposal is often non-sustainable. Landfill gas can be burned either directly for heat or to generate electricity for public consumption. Landfill gas contains approximately 50% methane, the gas found in natural gas. Land fill gas can be easily purified and then fed into the natural gas grid.

If landfill gas is not harvested, it escapes into the atmosphere: this is undesirable because methane is a greenhouse gas with much more global warming potential than carbon dioxide (Keppler *et al.*, 2009).

Over a time span of 100 years, one ton of methane produces the same greenhouse gas (GHG) effect as 21 tons of CO_2.

When methane burns, it produces carbon dioxide in the ratio 1:1—

$$CH_4 + 2O_2 = CO_2 + 2H_2O$$

So, by harvesting and burning landfill gas, its global warming potential is reduced a factor of 23, in addition to providing energy for heat and power. It was proved that living plants also produce methane. The amount is 10 to 100 times greater than that produced by dead plants in an aerobic environment but does not increase global warming because of the carbon cycle.

Anaerobic digestion can be used as a waste management strategy to reduce the amount of waste sent to landfill and generate methane, or biogas. Any form of biomass can be used in anaerobic digestion and will breakdown to produce methane, which can be harvested and burned to generate heat, power or to power certain automotive vehicles. A current project for a 1.6 MW landfill power plant is projected to provide power for 880 homes. It is estimated that this will eliminate 3,187 tons of methane and directly eliminate 8.756 tons of carbon dioxide release per year. This is the same as removing 12,576 cars from the road, or planting 15,606 trees, or not using 359 rail cars of coal per year.

The help of insects might be required to make a biofuel like bioethanol commercially viable, according to an entomologist (Washington). Michael Scharf, entomologist at the University of Florida, Gainesville and his colleague Aurélien Tartar informed how enzymes produced by both termites and the microorganisms that inhabit their gut—known as symbionts—could help to produce ethanol from non-edible plant material such as straw and wood.

Through millions and millions of years of evolution, termites and their symbionts have acquired highly specialised enzymes that work together to efficiently convert wood and other plant materials into simple sugars. These enzymes are of the most value to bioethanol production.

Current bioethanol production processes tend to use edible plant materials, such as starch from corn (maize) and sugar from sugar cane, which contain easily accessible sugar molecules that can be fermented to produce ethanol.

Using food crops to produce ethanol has proved highly controversial, with bioethanol being blamed for much of the recent rises in food prices.

The non-edible parts of many plants also contain a large number of sugar molecules, which could potentially be used to produce ethanol. But the problem is that these sugar molecules are far less accessible. This is because they are locked up within a substance known as lignocellulose, which provides structural support for plant cell walls (Tokuda *et al.*, 2007).

Breaking this substance up into its component sugar molecules is far from easy. One approach involves pretreating the lignocellulose by heating it in combination with acids or bases and then exposing the pretreated material to various enzymes. Another approach is very fine grinding followed by enzymatic treatment.

Termites, on the other hand, do not seem to have too much trouble digesting wood and other lignocellulosic materials into their component sugars, as many homeowners can attest.

The termite appears to favour the fine grinding approach in combination with its own unique set of enzymes. These enzymes are secreted by both termites and the symbionts that colonise their gut, and act on the lignocellulose that has been chewed to very small particles by the termite (Brune *et al.*, 2006).

Despite the small size of the termite gut and the difficulty in analysing its contents, a few research groups have attempted to study what Scharf and Tartar call the termite digestome. This is the pool of genes, both termite and symbiont, that code for the enzymes that breakdown and digest lignocellulosic material. Using a variety of genomic and proteomic techniques, these groups have managed to identify a number of the main enzymes, many of which could prove useful for producing ethanol (Brennan *et al.*, 2004).

This has already provided strong preliminary evidence that the enzymes produced by the termites and their symbionts tend to work collaboratively, with the lignocellulosic material having to be partially digested by termite enzymes before it can be further digested by symbiont enzymes. The study is scheduled for publication in biofuels, bioproducts and biorefining (Kambhampati *et al.*, 2000) (Fig. 8.1).

The **termites** are a group of eusocial insects usually classified at the taxonomic rank of order **Isoptera**. Termites are sometimes called "white ants", though they are not closely related to true ants. Along with ants and some bees and wasps which are all placed in the separate order Hymenoptera, termites divide labour among gender lines, produce overlapping generations and take care of young collectively. Termites mostly

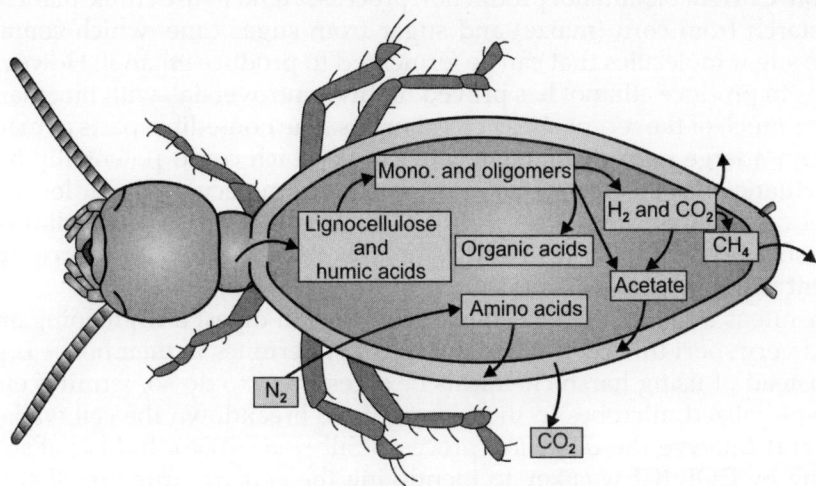

Fig. 8.1: Termites

feed on dead plant material, generally in the form of wood, leaf litter, soil, or animal dung, and about 10% of the estimated 4,000 species are economically significant as pests that can cause serious structural damage to buildings, crops or plantation forests. Termites are major detritivores, particularly in the subtropical and tropical regions, and their recycling of wood and other plant matter is of considerable ecological importance (Brune *et al.*, 1995).

As eusocial insects, termites live in colonies that, at maturity, number from several hundred to several million individuals. Colonies use a decentralised, self-organised systems of activity guided by swarm intelligence to exploit food sources and environments that could not be available to any single insect acting alone. A typical colony contains nymphs (semi-mature young), workers, soldiers, and reproductive individuals of both genders, sometimes containing several egg-laying queens (Davies *et al.*, 2002).

BIOFUELS FROM TERMITES

There are many directions that the science can now head. "First, we now have the ability to produce and test individual enzymes for their competency and roles in lignocellulose degradation. Once we identify major players (from termites and symbionts), we can test combinations that may have applications in making bioethanol production more feasible from existing feedstocks, and may be even other feedstocks that are not on their radar screens yet." (McHardy *et al.*, 2007).

Their digestome analysis could also be applied to other insects that feed on woody material, such as wood-boring beetles, and certain wasps and flies. Enzymes produced by both termites and the microorganisms that inhabit their gut could help to produce biofuel from non-edible plant material such as straw and wood. Through millions and millions years of evolution, termites and their symbionts have acquired highly specialised enzymes that work together to efficiently convert wood and other plant materials into simple sugars. These enzymes are of the most value to bioethanol production. Current bioethanol production processes tend to use edible plant materials, such as starch from corn (maize) and sugar from sugar cane, which contain easily accessible sugar molecules that can be fermented to produce ethanol. However, using food crops to produce ethanol has proved highly controversial, with bioethanol being blamed for much of the recent rises in food prices. The non-edible parts of many plants also contain a large number of sugar molecules, which could potentially be used to produce ethanol. But the problem is that these sugar molecules are far less accessible. This is because they are locked up within a substance known as lignocellulose, which provides structural support for plant cell walls. Breaking this substance up into its component sugar molecules is far from easy (Tringe, 2005).

The termite is a remarkable machine. Termites can digest a frightening amount of wood in a very short time, as anyone who has had termites in their house is painfully aware. Instead of using harsh chemicals or excess heat to do so, termites employ an array of specialized microbes in their hindguts to breakdown the cell walls of plant material and catalyze the digestion process (Gill *et al.*, 2006). Industrial-scale DNA sequencing by DOE JGI was key to identifying the genetic structures that comprise the tools that termites use.

It is in process to discover the metabolic pathways generated by these structures to figure out how nature digests plant materials. The novel enzymes can be synthesize discovered through this project to accelerate the delivery of the next generation of cellulosic biofuels.

While termites have been the subject of keen scientific study for more than a century, the precise identity and role of the microbes from their digestive tract remained a mystery. With this new work, the symbiotic orchestration of these compartmentalized, complex microbial communities required for wood digestion is now coming to light (Qi, 2005).

Like cows, termites have a series of stomachs, each harboring a distinct community of microbes under precisely defined conditions. These bugs within bugs are tasked with particular steps along the conversion pathway of woody polymers to sugars that can then be fermented into fuels such as ethanol. The mandibles of the insect chomp the wood into bits, but the real work is conducted in the dark recesses of the belly, where the enzymatic juices exuded by microbes attack and deconstruct the cellulose and hemicellulose, which, along with lignin, are the basic building blocks of wood (Odelson *et al.*, 1985).

The genomic sequencing and analysis of the termite gut microbes by the US Department of Energy Joint Genome Institute (DOE JGI), the California Institute of Technology, Verenium Corporation (formerly Diversa), a biofuels company, INBio, the National Biodiversity Institute of Costa Rica, and the IBM Thomas J. Watson Research Center, are highlighted in the November 22 edition of the journal Nature.

The tiny insects that gave up their stomach contents to advance the frontiers of science were isolated on a safari into the rainforest of Costa Rica, the world's geographic hotbed of biodiversity for termites, by co-author Jared Leadbetter of Cal Tech, first author Falk Warnecke of DOE JGI's Microbial Ecology Program, and members of Verenium and INBio. Traipsing through the jungle, the team came upon a massive, tumor-like nest of termites clinging to an otherwise nondescript tree. With a flick of a machete, the contents of this dense network of tunnels forged from wood waste were revealed, along with a frenzy of higher termites from the genus Nasutitermes, which are only about the size of the date imprinted on a penny (Tringe, 2005).

About 71 million letters of fragmented genetic code were elaborated and computationally reassembled, to tease out the identities of the microbial players in the mixture and the metabolic profile of the enzymes that they produce. From this reconstructed liquid puzzle emerged the identities of a dozen different phyla broad groupings of microbial life forms.

An analysis revealed that the hindgut is dominated by two major bacterial lineages, treponemes and fibrobacters (Phil Hugenholtz, DOE JGI's Microbial Ecology). Treponemes have long been recognized in the termite gut due to their distinctive cork-screw shape, but fibrobacters were an exciting new find, because they have relatives in the cow rumen known to degrade cellulose. The termite fibrobacters and treponemes could be directly linked to enzymes capable of breaking down wood. However, fibrobacters are specialists in this regard and do not appear to participate in sugar fermentation, leaving that to the treponemes. Termite can also be said as a mobile miniature bioreactor (Vignais et al., 2004).

In the termite gut compartment alone, more than 500 genes related to the enzymatic deconstruction of cellulose and hemicellulose were identified by Hugenholtz and colleagues. Adapting these findings for an industrial-scale system is far from easy.

Termites can efficiently convert milligrams of lignocellulose into fermentable sugars in their tiny bioreactor hindguts. There should be some work on scaling up this process so that biomass factories can produce biofuels more efficiently and economically. To get there, we must define the set of genes with key functional attributes for the breakdown of cellulose, and this study represents an essential step along that path (Pester et al., 2007).

The termite hindgut whodunit builds upon "metagenomic" research, where genetic material is isolated, identified, and characterized directly from environmental samples, providing a profile of a particular (often extreme) ecological niche. This includes glimpses into such diverse slices of the biosphere as acid mine drainage, a gutless worm, farm soil, submerged whalebones, and sewage sludge.

Currently among the scores of projects Tammar wallaby forestomach, the Asian longhorned beetle gut, and other exotic species promise to be treasure troves of enzymes involved in cellulose deconstruction.

Researchers at Berkeley Lab's Joint Genome Institute, California Institute of Technology, and Verenium Corporation have discovered and sequenced over 300 microbes in the hindgut of a Costa Rican termite and identified over 600 genes that encode for enzymes that may play a role in the termite's conversion of wood mass to sugars. The enzymes could enable more efficient strategies for the production of liquid biofuels from a variety of feedstocks (Pester et al., 2007).

Termites are extremely successful at degrading plant biomass including wood and grass, and are, therefore, important sources of biochemical catalysts that might be used in industrial lignocellulose degradation. Recent research has supported the idea that symbiotic microbes found in the termite hindgut play a direct role in cellulose and xylan hydrolysis—the step that has been the economic bottleneck in man-made systems that convert cellulose to biofuels. In fact, these microbes are so efficient that they are capable of producing about 2 liters of hydrogen from fermentation of a typical sheet of paper.

A relatively small set of fungal enzymes is used today for the hydrolysis of cellulose to simple sugars for subsequent fermentation, but the process is energy intensive, may involve toxic chemicals for pretreatment, and no discernable pathway exists for significant improvement. An optimized cocktail of the new termite-microbe enzymes could lead to conversion that is both energy and chemically efficient.

The Berkeley Lab-CIT-Verenium research is the first system-wide gene analysis of a microbial community specialized towards plant lignocellulose degradation. It revealed that the hindgut of the "higher" Nasutitermes species contains a broad diversity of bacteria representing 12 phyla and 216 phylotypes, and is dominated by two major bacterial lineages, treponemes and fibrobacters. While treponemes have been known to exist in the termite gut, fibrobacters are an exciting new find because they have relatives in the cow rumen known to degrade cellulose and are specialists in this regard.

Berkeley Labs, scientists are continuing research on the enzymes in order to define the set of genes with key functional attributes for the breakdown of cellulose and to determine metabolic pathways involved in the processes.

TYPES OF MICROBES PRESENT IN TERMITES GUT

Strict anaerobic culture techniques were used to quantitate heterotrophic bacteria present in hindguts of *Reticulitermes flavipes* (Warnecke, 2007) of a total of 344 isolates, 66.3% were streptococci that were always obtained regardless of the origin of termites, their developmental stage or caste, or their length of captivity. Most of the remaining isolates were strains of *Bacteroides* and *Enterobacteriaceae*. A small percentage were strains of *Lactobacillus*, *Fusobacterium*, and unidentified anaerobic Gram-positive rods. Recovery of bacteria from worker hindguts was 13.0% of the direct microscopic count. Isolations performed aerobically failed to reveal strict aerobes. Attempts to isolate cellulolytic bacteria were uniformly unsuccessful. Of 145 streptococcal strains isolated from freshly collected termites, almost all were *Streptococcus lactis* and *S. cremoris*. *Enterobacteriaceae* isolates from the same termite specimens were indole-positive *Citrobacter*, citrate-negative *Citrobacter*, and *Enterobacter cloacae*. The possibility of in situ interspecies lactate transfer, between lactate producers (e.g. streptococci) and lactate fermenters (bacteroides).

Diet

Termites are generally grouped according to their feeding behaviour. Thus, the commonly used general groupings are subterranean, soil-feeding, drywood, dampwood, and grass-eating. Of these, subterraneans and drywoods are primarily responsible for damage to human-made structures.

All termites eat cellulose in its various forms as plant fibre. Cellulose is a rich energy source (as demonstrated by the amount of energy released, when wood is burned), but remains difficult to digest. Termites rely primarily upon symbiotic protozoa (metamonads) such as *Trichonympha*, and other microbes in their gut to digest the cellulose for them and absorb the end products for their own use. Gut protozoa, such as *Trichonympha*, in turn rely on symbiotic bacteria embedded on their surfaces to produce some of the necessary digestive enzymes. This relationship is one of the finest examples of mutualism among animals. Most so called "higher termites", especially in the family Termitidae, can produce their own cellulase enzymes. However, they still retain a rich gut fauna and primarily rely upon the bacteria. Due to closely related bacterial species, it is strongly presumed that the termites' gut flora are descended from the gut flora of the ancestral wood-eating cockroaches, like those of the genus *Cryptocercus*.

Some species of termite practice fungiculture. They maintain a 'garden' of specialized fungi of genus *Termitomyces*, which are nourished by the excrement of the insects. When the fungi are eaten, their spores pass undamaged through the intestines of the termites to complete the cycle by germinating in the fresh faecal pellets (Odelson *et al.*, 1985). They are also well known for eating smaller insects in a last resort environment.

TERMITES AS A SOURCE OF POWER

The US Department of Energy is researching ways to replace fossil fuels with renewable sources of cleaner energy, and termites are considered a possible way to reach this goal through metagenomics.

Termites may produce up to two litres of hydrogen from digesting a single sheet of paper, making them one of the planet's most efficient bioreactor (Tokuda *et al.*, 2007). Termites achieve this high degree of efficiency by exploiting the metabolic capabilities of about 200 different species of microbes that inhabit their hindguts. The microbial community in the termite gut efficiently manufactures large quantities of hydrogen; the complex lignocellulose polymers within wood are broken down into simple sugars by fermenting bacteria in the termite's gut, using enzymes that produce hydrogen as a byproduct. A second wave of bacteria uses the simple sugars and hydrogen to make the acetate the termite requires for energy. By sequencing the termite's microbial community, the DOE hopes to get a better understanding of these biochemical pathways. If it can be determined which enzymes are used to create hydrogen, and which genes produce them, this process could potentially be scaled up with bioreactors to generate hydrogen from woody biomass, such as poplar, in commercial quantities (Delucchi *et al.*, 2008).

Sceptics regard this as unlikely to become a carbon-neutral commercial process due to the energy inputs required to maintain the system. For decades, researchers have sought to house termites on a commercial scale (like worm farms) to breakdown woody debris and paper, but funding has been scarce and the problems of developing a continuous process that does not disrupt the termites' homeostasis have not been overcome (Brune, 2000).

Ecology

Ecologically, termites are important in nutrient recycling, habitat creation, soil formation and quality and, particularly the winged reproductives, as food for countless predators. The role of termites in hollowing timbers and thus providing shelter and increased wood surface areas for other creatures is critical for the survival of a large number of timber-inhabiting species. Larger termite mounds play a role in providing a habitat for plants and animals, especially on plains in Africa that are seasonally inundated by a rainy season, providing a retreat above the water for smaller animals and birds, and a growing medium for woody shrubs with root systems that cannot withstand inundation for several weeks. In addition, scorpions, lizards, snakes, small mammals, and birds live in abandoned or weathered mounds, and aardvarks dig substantial caves and burrows in them, which then become homes for larger animals such as hyenas and mongooses (Bignelle *et al.*, 2000).

As detrivores, termites clear away leaf and woody litter and so reduce the severity of the annual bush fires in African savannas, which are not as destructive as those in Australia and the USA.

Globally, termites are found roughly between 50 degrees North and South, with the greatest biomass in the tropics and the greatest diversity in tropical forests and Mediterranean shrublands. Termites are also considered to be a major source of atmospheric methane, one of the prime greenhouse gases. Termites have been common since at least the Cretaceous period. Termites also eat bone and other parts of carcasses, and their traces have been found on dinosaur bones from the middle Jurassic in China (Tokuda, 2007).

STUDIES DONE ON TERMITES

The hard part in producing cellulosic ethanol is obtaining the metabolic intermediates from things like wood, but that's the problem the termites have solved. Cellulose is a fibrous complex carbohydrate that makes up plant cell walls. Biofuels made from cellulosic biomass, including cornstalks, woodchips, perennial grasses, and weeds such as switchgrass, could provide an alternative to corn-derived ethanol, which requires a large amount of energy to produce. Breaking down cellulose into simple sugars that can be fermented into ethanol is currently a complex, inefficient, and expensive process. Scientists are searching for new enzymes that can more efficiently breakdown the hardy molecule and allow the production process to compete with corn-based ethanol (Ohkuma *et al.*,1999).

STUDY OF TERMITES GUT BY METAGENOMIC METHODS

Jared Leadbetter, a microbiologist at Caltech, and his colleagues collected *Nasutitermes* termites from Costa Rica and isolated DNA from the microbial contents of part of their digestive tract. Scientists had previously theorized that these termite's wood-digesting powers come primarily from the microbes that live in their gut. Using a metagenomics approach, researchers sequenced and analyzed the genomic material from many different types of bacteria, searching for particular sequences known from other studies to be linked to the ability to breakdown cellulose. They identified nearly 1,000 candidate genes for glycohydrolases—enzymes that breakdown complex plant carbohydrates, such as cellulose.

Researches are still going on that how termites, which derive virtually all their nutrients from woond, breakdown the material so efficiently. Termites have been turning wood into their own biofuel for 200 million years.

The next step should be to figure out exactly what the different enzymes do. The functional analysis has to be done. It is in process to access the solid cellulose matrix, a process that requires specific mixtures of enzymes.

Experimental studies are going in the wood-digesting ability of some of the newly identified microbial enzymes, as well as for combinations of enzymes that work together synergistically. Microbial genes from the termite gut already appear to have several enzymes from a class known to be particularly powerful, as well as a wide variety of accessory enzymes necessary for the digestion process.

The termite gut microbial genome is likely to contain more genomic bounty. The researchers found 34 groups of genes with unknown function, including one specific sequence identified in a dozen other cellulose-digesting bacteria. Enzymes produced by termites can help to produced biofuel.

A new research has explored the possibilities of how enzymes produced by both termites and the microorganisms that inhabit their gut could help to produce biofuel from non-edible plant material such as straw and wood. Michael Scharf, an assistant professor of entomology at the University of Florida, Gainesville, and his colleague Aurelien Tartar undertook the research (Scarf, 2008).

Through millions and millions of years of evolution, termites and their symbionts have acquired highly specialised enzymes that work together to efficiently convert wood and other plant materials into simple sugars. These enzymes are of the most value to bioethanol production. Current bioethanol production processes tend to use edible plant materials, such as starch from corn (maize) and sugar from sugar cane, which contain easily accessible sugar molecules that can be fermented to produce ethanol.

However, using food crops to produce ethanol has proved highly controversial, with bioethanol being blamed for much of the recent rises in food prices. The non-edible parts of many plants also contain a large number of sugar molecules, which could potentially be used to produce ethanol. Converting plant lignocellulosic biomass to simple sugars for fermentation into biofuels, and hydrogen. Promises to be more energy and chemically efficient than the fungal enzymes currently in use. Combinations of the enzymes could be optimized for a particular feedstock.

Nanotechnology Makes Biofuel Development a Cost-effective and 'Green' Process

Research at Louisiana Tech University in the US has come out with nanotechnology processes that can make the development of biofuels cost-effective and also easy on the environment. Biofuels will play an important part in sustainable fuel and energy production solutions for the future.

A country's appetite for fuel, however, cannot be satisfied with traditional crops such as sugar cane or corn alone. Emerging technologies are allowing cellulosic biomass (wood, grass, stalks) to also be converted into ethanol.

Cellulosic ethanol does not compete with food production and has the potential to decrease greenhouse gas (GHG) emissions by 86% over that of today's fossil fuels. Current techniques for corn ethanol only reduce greenhouse gases by 19%.

The nanotechnology processes developed at Louisiana Tech University can immobilize the expensive enzymes used to convert cellulose to sugars, allowing them to be reused several times over and, thus significantly reducing the overall cost of the process.

Savings estimate range from approximately 32 million dollars for each cellulosic ethanol plant to a total of 7.5 billion dollars, if a federally-established goal of 16 billion gallons of cellulosic ethanol is achieved. This process can easily be applied in large-scale commercial environments and can immobilize a wide variety or mixture of enzymes for production.

ADVANTAGES OF BIOFUELS

The aim of all biofuels is to be carbon neutral. They reduce greenhouse gas emissions when compared to conventional transport fuels. In reality, biofuels are not carbon neutral simply because it requires energy to grow the crops and convert them into fuel. The amount of fuel used during this production (to power machinery, to transport crops, etc.) does have a large impact on the overall savings achieved by biofuels (Tringe, 2005).

However, biofuels still prove to be substantially more environment-friendly than their alternatives (Lal, 2005).

In fact, according to a technique called Life Cycle Analysis (LCA), first generation biofuels can save up to 60% of carbon emissions compared to fossil fuels. Second generation biofuels offer carbon emission savings up to 80%.

Another advantage of biofuels is that they save drivers money. The UK Government in particular has introduced many incentives to drivers of 'green cars' based on emissions — with reduced taxation dependent on how environment-friendly the vehicle is. With petrol prices on the rise, replacing petroleum with a renewable energy source should also offer significant savings at the pump in the long term, particularly when biofuels are more readily available. (Farrell, *et al.*, 2006).

There are arguments too that biofuels are helping to tackle poverty around the world. For example, the Overseas Development Institute has pointed to wider economic growth and increased employment opportunities along with the positive effect on energy prices, as reasons to back biofuel production. This is debated due to the pressures it places on agricultural resources but biodiesel could be a long-term solution as it uses simpler technology and lower transportation costs alongside increased labour (Fearnside *et al.*, 2000).

DISADVANTAGES OF BIOFUELS

- **Biodiversity** A fear among environmentalists is that by adapting more land to produce crops for biofuels, more habitats will be lost for animals and wild plants. It is feared, e.g. some Asian countries will sacrifice their rainforests to build more oil plantations.

- **The food vs fuel debate** Another concern is that if biofuels become lucrative for farmers, they may grow crops for biofuel production instead of food production. Less food production will increase prices and cause a rise in inflation. It is hoped that this can be countered by second generation biofuels which use waste biomass — though again, this will impact the habitat of many organisms. The impact is particularly high in developing countries and it is estimated that around 100 million people are at risk due to the food price increases (Righelato *et al.*, 2007).

- **Carbon emissions** Most LCA investigations show that the burning of biofuels substantially reduces greenhouse gas emissions, when compared to petroleum and diesel. However, in 2007 a study was published by scientists from Britain, the USA, Germany and Austria which reported the burning of rapeseed or corn can contribute as much to nitrous oxide emissions than cooling through fossil fuel savings (Guo *et al.*, 2000).

- **Non-sustainable biofuel production** Many first generation biofuels are not sustainable. It is necessary to create sustainable biofuel production that does not affect food production, and does not cause environmental problems.

- The production of non-sustainable biofuels has been criticised in reports by the UN. As a result, many governments have switched their support towards sustainable biofuels, and alternatives such as hydrogen and compressed air (Guo *et al.*, 2000).

Barriers

Ethanol supply is constrained by arable land availability. Competition with food production for land use could drive possible increases in both ethanol and food prices (already occurring in the sugar market). Ethanol markets still have a regional structure. Transport of biomass remains a logistics barrier that limits the size of ethanol production plants and economies of scale. A more liberalised market would create opportunities and incentives for producers in emerging economies especially Brazil, India, and Thailand. Transfer of advanced agricultural practices to developing countries could considerably help (Searchinger *et al.*, 2008).

Conversely, producing more biofuels from conventional feedstocks could conflict with conservation of biodiversity and call for increased amounts of water, pesticides and fertilisers, thus raising sustainability issues. In scenarios having 25% of transport fuels derived from biomass, the use of fertilisers increases by about 40%. On a fuel-cycle basis, ethanol, with its high vapour pressure, reduces NO_2 and volatile organic compound (VOC) emissions but this is partly offset from increased N_2O emission from increased use of nitrogenous fertilisers (Hill *et al.*, 2006).

Developing cost-effective ethanol production from lignocellulose via enzymatic hydrolysis would, therefore, increase the variety and availability of feedstocks and hence expand the production of biofuels. Other ethanol drawbacks include miscibility with water, aldehyde emissions, compatibility issues with some plastics or metals (Al-alloys, brass, zinc, lead) and high latent vapourisation heat (cold start issues). Ethanol use in compression ignition engines needs additives due to the low cetane number and is impractical (Howarth *et al.*, 2005).

Biodiesel production depends on feedstock and land availability even more than bioethanol production. The Fischer-Tropsch technology and other advanced processes hold the potential to increase biofuels production basis (Howarth *et al.*, 2005).

NEW RESEARCH PROMISES BOOST TO BIOFUEL PRODUCTION

Scientists in Nevada have found a new and environment-friendly source of biodiesel– "chicken feather meal", a delightful material that consists of chicken feathers, blood, and innards made from the 11 billion pounds of poultry industry waste that accumulates annually in the US alone.

Biofuels continue to steal the spotlight when it comes to the search for a renewable, environment-friendly replacement for crude oil. While that's understandable, when considering the transport industry, but crude oil is also used in the production of conventional plastics and chemical products such as fertilizers and solvents. Now chemists have learned how to convert plant biomass directly into a chemical building block that cannot only be used to produce fuel, but also plastics, polyester and industrial chemicals cheaply and efficiently (Nepstad *et al.*, 2007).

Running vehicles on biofuels such as ethanol reduces CO_2 emissions and offers a way to lessen the world's reliance on oil. While this sounds great from an environmental perspective, the energy required to produce the biofuel and the land clearing for crops that can result means biofuels are not necessarily the environment-friendly solution they initially appear to be (Stern et al., 2007).

Recognizing this, researchers have analyzed the best way to maximize the "miles per acre" from biomass and discovered that the far more efficient option is to convert the biomass to electricity, rather than ethanol. Scientists at the Singapore-based Institute of Bioengineering and Nanotechnology (IBN) have made an unprecedented breakthrough in transforming carbon dioxide, a common greenhouse gas, into methanol, a widely used form of industrial feedstock and clean-burning biofuel. Using "organocatalysts", researchers activated carbon dioxide in a mild and non-toxic process to produce the more useful chemical compound (Nordhaus et al., 2007).

While there are plenty of alternative fuel prospects floating around, a key factor in the widespread adoption of such fuels is whether or not they are economical. A team of New York based researchers have developed the first economical, Eco-friendly process to convert algae oil into biodiesel fuel—a discovery they predict could one day lead to US independence from petroleum as a fuel (O'Hare et al., 2009).

PRACTICAL PERFORMANCES AFTER USING BIOFUEL

Air New Zealand has successfully undertaken the world's first commercial aviation test flight using the second-generation biofuel jatropha.

Green Flight International has set another green-aviation record, this time flying a Jet across the US using environment-friendly biofuel.

BioJet 1 completed the flight from Reno, Nevada to Leesburg, Florida in just over 11 hours at altitudes ranging from 13,000 to 17,000 feet. While 1,776 miles where flown on 100% biofuel, a 50/50 mix of biofuel and standard jet fuel was used for the remainder of the 2,486 journey in order to compare performance data and also demonstrate the ability to blend these fuel types (Stavins et al., 2005).

REFERENCES

1. Adler PR, Del Grosso S J, Parton W J. Life-cycle assessment of net greenhouse-gas flux for bioenergy cropping systems. *Ecol. Appl.,* 17, 675–691; 2007.

2. Brune, A. In: Drowkin M, Falkow S, Rosenberg E, et al. (eds). *The Prokaryotes*; Springer, New York. 1:439–474; 2006.

3. Brennan Y et al. Unusual microbial xylanases from insect guts. *Appl Environ Microbiol* 70, 3609–3617 2004.

4. Brune A, Emerson, D, Breznak JA. The termite gut microflora as an oxygen sink: microelectrode determination of oxygen and pH gradients in guts of lower and higher termites. *Appl. Environ. Microbiol.* 61, 2681–2687; 1995.

5. Brune A, Friedrich M. Microecology of the termite gut: structure and function on a microscale. *Curr. Opin. Microbiol.* 3, 263–269; 2000.

6. Breznak, J. A. and Brune, A. Role of microorganisms in the digestion of lignocelluloses in termites. *Annu. Rev. Entomol.* 39, 453–487 (1994).

7. Breznak, J. A. and Switzer, J. M. Acetate synthesis from H_2 plus CO_2 by termite gut microbes. Appl. Environ. Microbiol. 52, 623–630 (1986).

8. Bignell, D. and Eggleton, P. *Termites: Evolution, Sociality, Symbioses, Ecology, eds.* Abe, T., Bignell, D. E. and Higashi, M. (Kluwer Academic,Dordrecht, The Netherlands), pp. 363–388 (2000).

9. Davies, G. J. and Henrissat, B. Structural enzymology of carbohydrate-active enzymes: implications for the post-genomic era. *Biochem. Soc.* Trans. 30, 291–297 (2002).

10. Delucchi, M.A. Important Issues in life-cycle Analysis of CO_2- Equivalent Greenhouse-Gas Emissions from Biofuels." Presented at "Workshop on Measuring and Modeling the Lifecycle GHG Impacts of Transportation Fuels," Berkeley, CA, July (2008).

11. Farrell, Alexander E., Richard Plevin, Brian Turner, Andrew Jones, Michael O'Hare, and Daniel Kammen. "Ethanol Can Contribute to Energy and Environmental Goals." *Science* 311: 506–508. (2006)

12. Fearnside, P.M., D.A. Lashof, P. Moura-Costa. "Accounting for Time in Mitigating Global Warming Through Land-Use Change and Forestry." *Mitigation and Adaptation Strategies for Global Change* 5 (3): 239–270. (2000)

13. Farrell, A. E., Plevin, R. J., Turner, B. T., Jones, A. D., O'Hare, M., and Kammen, D. M.: EthanolCan Contribute to Energy and Environmental Goals, Science, 311, 506–508, (2006).

14. Gill, S. R. et al. Metagenomic analysis of the human distal gut microbiome. *Science* 312, 1355–1359 (2006).

15. Guo, J., C. Hepburn, R.S. J. Tol, D. Anthoff. "Discounting and the social cost of carbon: a closer look at uncertainty." *Envir. Sci. and Pol.* 9 (3): 205–216 (2006)

16. Hill, Jason, Erik Nelson, David Tilman, Stephen Polasky, and Douglas Tiffany. "Environmental, economic, and energetic costs and benefits of biodiesel and ethanol biofuels." *Proc. of the Natl. Acad. of Sci.* 103 (30): 11206–11210 (2006)

17. Howarth, R.B. "Against High Discount Rates." *Advances in the Economics of Environmental Research* 5: 103–124. (2005)

18. Hill, J., Nelson, E., Tilman, D., Polasky, S., and Tiffany, D.: Environmental, economic, and energetic costs and benefits of biodiesel and ethanol biofuels. *Proc. Natl. Acad. Sci.*, 103,11 206–11 210, (2006).

19. IPCC:IPCC Guidelines for National Greenhouse Gas Inventories, prepared by the National Greenhouse Gas Inventories Programme, edited by: Eggleston, H. S., Buendia, L., Miwa, K., Ngara, T., and Tanabe, K., Volume 4, Chapter 11, N_2O emissions from managed soils, and CO2 emissions from lime and urea application, IGES, Hayama, Japan, (2006).

20. Kambhampati, S. and Eggleton, P. in Termites: Evolution, Sociality, Symbioses, Ecology (eds Abe, T. Bignell, D. E. and Higashi, M.) 1–24 (Kluwer Academic, Dordrecht (2000).

21. Lal, R.: World crop residues production and implications of its use as a bio-fuel. *Environment International*, 31, 575–584 (2005).

22. Marshall, A. T. *Bioenergy from Waste: A Growing Source of Power, Waste Management World Magazine April*, p34–37 (2007)

23. McHardy, A. C., Martin, H. G., Tsirigos, A., Hugenholtz, P. and Rigoutsos, I. Accurate phylogenetic classification of variable-length DNA fragments. *Nat. Methods* 4, 63–72 (2007).

24. Nepstad, D.C. C.M. Stickler, B. Soares- Filho, and F. Merry. "Interactions among Amazon land use, forests and climate: prospects for a near-term forest tipping point" *Phil. Trans. R. Soc.* B, DOI: 10.1098/rstb.0026 (2008).

25. Nordhaus, W'. "Critical Assumptions in the Stern Review on Climate Change." *Science* 317: 201–202 (2007).

26. O'Hare, M., R.J. Plevin, J.I. Martin, A.D. Jones, A. Kendall, and E. Hopson. "Proper accounting for time increases crop-based biofuels' greenhouse gas deficit versus petroleum." *Environ. Res. Lett.* 4: 024001 (7 pp.) (2009)

27. Odelson, D. A. and Breznak, J. A. Nutrition and growth characteristics of Trichomitopsis termopsidis, a cellulolytic protozoan from termites. *Appl. Environ.Microbiol.* 49, 614–621 (1985).

28. Ohkuma, M., Noda, S. and Kudo, T. Phylogenetic diversity of nitrogen fixation genes in the symbiotic microbial community in the gut of diverse termites. *Appl. Environ. Microbiol.* 65, 4926–4934 (1999).

29. Pester, M. and Brune, A. Hydrogen is the central free intermediate during lignocellulose degradation by termite gut symbionts. *ISME J.* 1, 551–565 (2007).

30. Pester, M. and Brune, A. Expression profiles of fhs (FTHFS) genes support the hypothesis that spirochaetes dominate reductive acetogenesis in the hindgut of lower termites. *Environ. Microbiol.* 8, 1261–1270 (2006).

31. Prather, M., Ehhalt, D. 2001. Atmospheric chemistry and greenhouse gases, edited by:Houghton, J. T., Ding, Y., Griggs, D. J., et al.: In: *Climate Change: The Scientific Basis*, pp. 239–287, Cambridge University Press, Cambridge, UK, (2001).

32. Pu, Yunqiao; Dongcheng Zhang, Preet M. Singh and Arthur J. Ragauskas "The new forestry biofuels sector". *Biofuels, Bioproducts and Biorefining (BioFPR)* 2 (1): 58–73 (2007)

33. Keppler F, John T. G. Hamilton, Marc Bra, and Thomas Röckmann "Methane emissions from terrestrial plants under aerobic conditions". *Nature*, 439: 187–191. (2006).

34. Kambhampati, S. and Eggleton, P. In: *Termites: Evolution, Sociality, Symbioses, Ecology* (eds Abe, T. Bignell, D. E. and Higashi, M.) 1–24 (Kluwer Academic, Dordrecht (2000).

35. Qi, M. et al. Novel molecular features of the fibrolytic intestinal bacterium Fibrobacter intestinalis not shared with Fibrobacter succinogenes as determined by suppressive subtractive hybridization. *J. Bacteriol.*, 187: 3739–3751 (2005).

36. Richards, K.R. "The Time Value of Carbon in Bottom-Up Studies." *Critical Reviews in Environmental Science and Technology* 27 (special): S279–s292 (1997)

37. Righelato, R., and D.V. Spracklen. "Carbon Mitigation by Biofuels or by Saving and Restoring Forests?" *Science* 317 (5840): 902 (2007)

38. Scharf M.E, Tartar. M.A . *Inset Biochemistry and Molecular Biology* 10.1002/bbb.107, 2008.

39. Searchinger, T., R. Heimlich, R. A. Houghton, F. Dong, A. Elobeid, J. Fabiosa, S. Tokgoz, D. Hayes, and T.-H. Yu. "Use of U.S. Croplands for Biofuels Increases Greenhouse Gases Through Emissions from Land Use Change." *Science* 319 (5867): 1238–1240 (2008).

40. Stavins, R.N. and K.R. Richards. "The Cost of U.S. Forest-Based Carbon Sequestration." 40 pp. Prepared for the Pew Center on Global Climate Change (2005)

41. Stern, N. and C. Taylor. "Climate Change: Risk, Ethics, and the Stern Review." *Science* 317: 203–204 (2007)

42. Taylor, L. E. II et al. Complete cellulase system in the marine bacterium *Saccharophagus degradans* strain 2–40T. *J. Bacteriol.* 188, 3849–3861 (2006).

43. Tokuda, G. and Watanabe, H. Hidden cellulases in termites: revision of an old hypothesis. *Biol. Lett.* 3, 336–339 (2007).

44. Tokuda, G. et al. Major alteration of the expression site of endogenous cellulases in members of an apical termite lineage. *Mol. Ecol.* 13, 3219–3228 (2004).

45. Tringe, S. G. et al. Comparative metagenomics of microbial communities. *Science* 308, 554–557 (2005).

46. Venter, J. C. et al. Environmental genome shotgun sequencing of the Sargasso Sea. *Science* 304, 66–74 (2004).

47. Vignais, P. M. and Colbeau, A. Molecular biology of microbial hydrogenases. *Curr. Issues Mol. Biol.* 6, 159–188 (2004).

48. Warnecke, F. et al, "Metagenomic and Functional Analysis of Hindgut Microbiota of a Wood-Feeding Higher Termite,". *Nature*, 450, 560–565.) (2007)

49. Xie, G. et al. Genome sequence of the cellulolytic gliding bacterium Cytophaga hutchinsonii. *Appl. Environ. Microbiol.* 73, 3536–3546 (2007).

50. Zah, R., H. Boni, M. Gauch, R. Hischier, M. Lehmann, and P. Wager. "Life Cycle Assessment of Energy Productions: Environmental Assessment of Biofuels Executive Summary." *EMPA*, Switzerland. (2007).

9

Building Biodeteriorating Fungi and their Impacts on Human Health

Padma Singh • Mamta Chauhan

INTRODUCTION

Biodeterioration implies a change in the value of the material which makes the material less useful in aesthetic or utilitarian terms. Biodeterioration can be brought about by a variety of living organisms including insects, pests, microorganisms, etc. Materials, even when humid, do not provide a ready supply of nutrients, and microorganisms can invade these materials only if they have the capacity to breakdown constituents to give utilizable nutrients. The ability of organisms to breakdown constituents is due to elaboration of enzymes like cellulases and proteinases. A building, however, is a long lasting product compared with many other utility goods and different kinds of ageing and damage caused by several reasons may occur. There is different types of buildings and structures, and the performance of the whole building depends on many factors—materials, structures, coating, climate, environment, type of use, service, etc.

During the service life of buildings, natural ageing and eventual damage of materials due to different chemical, physical and biological processes can take place. Ageing of the materials is one aspect of the environmental processes and involves different chemical, mechanical and biological reactions of the materials biodeterioration, e.g. mould, decay and insect damage in buildings, is caused when moisture exceeds the tolerance of the structures which may be a critical factor for durability and usage of different building materials (Grant et. al. 1989, Hyvarinen et. al. 2002). The other abiotic factors like UV radiation and quality of substrate are also significant for the growth of organisms. Different organisms, e.g. bacteria, fungi and insects, can grow and live in the building materials; microbiologically clean building do not exist, as some contamination beings as early as during the construction phase (Leivo and Rantala 2008). The humidity (moisture) conditions connected with temperature and exposure time are the most factor for development of biological problems and damage in buildings. The overall functionality of building is important to keep in mind during design, construction and preparation of a building. The structure should be functional, and the ventilation and plumbing systems together with automation should support the overall functionality (Airaksinen et al. 2007).

Fungal colonization of interior surfaces occurs, when biodegradable materials are chronically damp or wet. If growth is extensive, the consequence can be a structural defect (e.g. fungi degrade the paper fiber surface of wallboard) or a health problem (e.g. allergic respiratory disease). Fungi will grow on damp/moist biodegradable construction and finishing materials. The primary environmental factor controlling the growth of fungi in buildings is moisture availability. Moisture can enter buildings from sources such as rainwater as pipe/sprinkler leaks. Moisture can also occur in building materials from less obvious sources involving water vapor migration and infiltration of humid outdoor air into the building envelope. Wind driven rain can enter the building envelope and saturate construction materials especially when roof and window flashing fails. Water that enters the building envelope should be removed by drainage to the outside or by collection of water vapor by the air-conditioning dehumidification cooling coil.

Construction defects in building envelopes where water drainage to the outside is blocked by mortar and other construction debris is common. Because of this defect, rain water that enter the envelope chronically drains into the occupied space. This results in wetting of paper fiber, gypsum board and flooring materials with subsequent fungal growth. In warm humid climates, condensation occurs on walls, ceilings, and floors, when their surface temperatures are cooled (by air conditioning) below the dew point temperature of the surrounding air. If warm, moist outdoor air infiltrates through envelope wall (in a negatively pressurized building) condensation or dampness occurs on cool surfaces (e.g. wallpaper, paper fiber, gypsum board). Fungi then colonize these surfaces. Ageing of the materials is often a result of different chemical reactions of the material. The abiotic factors like temperature, water and quality of substrate (nutrients, pH, water permeability) are also the more significant for the growth of organisms. In some cases, UV radiation, air movements and gases of air have effects on the ageing, but also on microbial growth. However, the effect of these factors is often indirect. Air circulation affects humidity conditions, particle accumulation and composition of air and surfaces.

Mould and Decay Problems in Buildings

Mould and decay problems in buildings are caused by moisture damage — water leakage, convection of damp air and moisture condensation, rising damp from the ground and moisture accumulation in the structure. In buildings, mould fungi cause problems in different structure and materials such as roofs, attics, basement, floors and walls.

Mould Fungi

The growth of mould fungi on materials on buildings is often an early indication of increased humidity or moisture levels, but the problems caused by fungi in buildings vary depending on the types of fungal attack. Problems caused by mould fungi are mainly discoloration, odor and health disadvantages. The typical mould fungi in water damaged finishing building are Ascomycetes fungi: *Alternaria, Penicillium, Fusarium,*

Aspergillus, Trichoderma, Acremonium species (Table 9.1). Mould fungi cause several problems in buildings—stains, smell, health problems, etc. Also in the sound buildings, however, mould growth can be found on facades, attics and crawl spaces, which are typical structures exposed to high humidity conditions and attacked by mould fungi (Viitanen, 1997).

Table 9.1: Selected mould fungi found in damp buildings

S. No.	Fungal species	Substrate	Possible metabolites	Potential health effect
1	Alternaria alternata	Moist window sills walls	Allergens	Asthma, allergy
2	Aspergillus versicolor	Damp wood wall paper glue	Mycotoxins, VOCs	Unknown
3	Aspergillus fumigatus	House dust, potting soil	Allergens	Asthma, rhinitis, pneumonitis
4	Cladosporium herbarum	Moist window sills, wood	Allergens	Asthma, allergy
5	Penicillium chrysogenum	Damp wall paper, behind paint	Mycotoxins	Unknown
6	Penicillium expansum	Damp wallpaper	Mycotoxins	Nephrotoxicity
7	Stachybotrys chartarum	Heavily wetted carpet, gypsum board	Mycotoxins	Dermatitis, mucosal irritation, immunosuppression

Decay Fungi

Three different decay types are classified and found also in buildings—brown rot, soft rot and white rot. Most of the brown rot and white rot fungi belong to *Basidiomycetes*, but some belong to *Ascomycetes*. Most of the soft rot fungi belong to *Ascomycetes*. In buildings suffering from excessive moisture loading, brown rot is the most common decay type. Among the typical brown rot fungi which cause the most serious damage in buildings in temperate climates are *Serpula lacrymans*(dry rot fungus). Especially the dry rot fungus *S. lacrymans*, which is able to transport water through mycelial strands from the source of moisture into the dry wood (Viitanen, 2000).

Fungi that Colonize Building Materials

A wide range of fungal species can normally be cultured from air and dust samples in all buildings, as spores are brought in the air, or tracked in by animals and occupants. Many of these will colonize building materials, if given the right conditions. *Aspergillus flaves, A. versicolor, Alternaria alternata, Rhizopus* sp., *Mucur* sp., *Penicillium* sp., *Fusarium* sp. *Trichoderma* sp (Fig. 9.1, colour plate 4).

Conditions that Encourage Growth

The species found on building materials depends on available moisture, temperature and found source, but primarily on moisture. Their growth on culture plates depends on the handling of sample, type of culture medium used, temperature and moisture

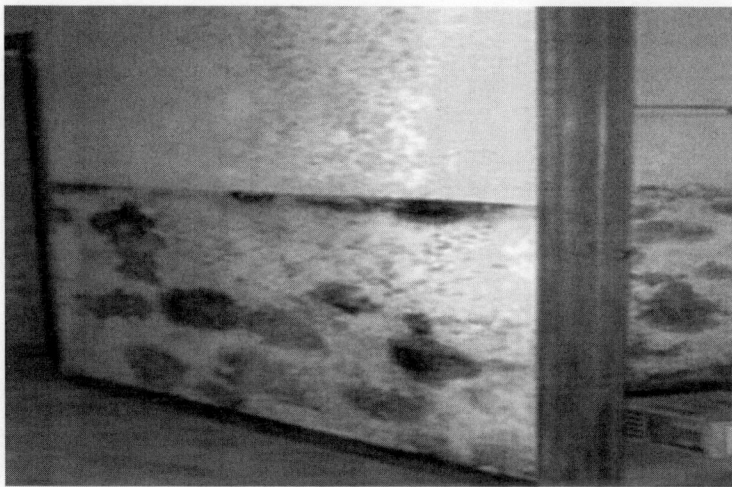

Fig. 9.1: Building deteriorating fungi

conditions during culturing, and competition between species on the culture plates. The primary factor in mold growth is available moisture in the substrate, which is measured as an equilibrium relative humidity at the surface where growth occurs, commonly expressed as water activity (aw). At an water activity of 0.65 (65% RH at the surface), no significant fungal growth can occur. Dump materials (aw 0.65 to 0.85) which are subject to biodeterioration can support growth of relatively xerophilic (dry-loving) fungi such as *Eurotium* sp., *Aspergillus versicolor*. Materials that are chronically wet (aw >0.9) are dominated by hydrophilic fungi such as *Ulocladium*, *Stachybutrys*, and *Fusarium* sp., etc. which are sometimes referred to as "signature flood fungi" (Morey et al, 2000; Morey, 1997).

MANAGEMENT OF BUILDING DAMAGES

Humidity and Moisture Control

In buildings, the performance of wood and other materials is greatly dependant on structural provisions. The main principal of structural protection is to eliminate or diminish the risk of fungal decay by designing and maintaining the constructions so that they remain constantly dry or are allowed to dry rapidly after wetting. The moisture content of wood should remain under 20–25%. RH of 80–90% is a critical humidity level for growth of mould fungi, but also temperature, exposure time and surface of materials are important factors. RH 90–95% is often critical level for the development of decay at 10–40°C. Water supports germination, hyphal growth and sporulation of fungi. Air humidity and microclimate is critical for sporulation, spore release and survival of spores. The major factors affecting the microclimate are moisture migration and accumulation in materials, composition, texture and surface quality of material, temperature, humidity, water condensation and air circulation. In buildings, the dry rot fungus, however, can transport water and cause more serious damage due to the extensive mycelial spread from a moisture source to dry wood.

Chemical Treatments to Protect Materials

The preservation of wood with chemicals is a conventional technique to add the durability of wood. Different types of chemicals has been used. Tar and creosote oils are very old preservatives. Tar oil is used for protection of shingle roofs, boats, fences, etc. Ochre paints are very permeable paints; oil paints are less permeable. Permeability of many modern acrylate paints is higher than that of oil paints or alkyl oil paints.

Heat treatment of wood is very popular topic in finland and in Europe at the moment. The basic of this technology is very old. Wood was fire treated already in ancient times.

STRUCTURE

Wet Rooms and Floors

In wet rooms, water is most often penetrated through inside surface or pipe leakage into the structures. Good water proofing is essential regardless of whether the building is made of stone or wood. The walls and floor must be water proof, which means joints and inlets must be carefully sealed. Good ventilation during and after use of the room removes moisture that places a stress on the surface in the room. If ventilation caps are closed, severe decay problems have been found. The ground-based floor is used in the old buildings. This type of floor is very sensitive for water damage and microbial growth. In the newer buildings, wooden beams are often based on concrete slab on ground. As insulation materials, moss, wood chips or mineral wool is most often used. This type of structure is often sensitive for moisture stress, and mould or decay damages has often been found due to water damage. Water proofing material, such as bitumen felt should be placed between wooden and concrete parts. In conjunction with repair, bricks or concrete blocks should be used to raise the wooden supporting rails of the wood floor above the level of the lower concrete slab. Water-proof material should also be placed between the brick or concrete block and the wooden structure. The wooden parts of interior walls should always be above the finished floor and insulated from the concrete below by means of strips of bitumen.

Indoor Air

Inside air quality, however, is primarily dependent on the ventilation system of a building. Regardless of what kind of ventilation system is used, it must be capable of exchanging a sufficient amount of air to prevent hazardous substances from accumulating indoors. This is very important especially in cold climate, and controlled air ventilation is needed to save the energy consumption. If the interior surface of a building is made of porous material, such as wood or construction sheeting, they may accumulate moisture and possibly other gaseous substances. This can affect the inside air quality.

Potential Health Effects

Recent large scale epidemiological studies have shown an association between adverse human health effects and dampness in buildings (Miller and Day, 1998). Further studies suggest that fungal exposure can exacerbate asthma symptoms, trigger allergic reactions, elicit an immune system response, cause invasive and opportunistic infections in humans, and may also cause toxic disease (Ponikav, 1999; IOM, 2000; Burge, 2000). Adverse health effects are associated with occupancy of buildings with moisture and mould damage. Mucormycosis is an uncommon, rapidly progressive fungal infection with a reputation for diagnostic difficulties, unsatisfactory treatment and a high mortality. Some fungi cause skin infections, including ringworm and athlete's foot. Inhalation of certain species can cause toxic reactions. Fungal infections that pose no threat to healthy individuals can be fetal to those suffering immunodeficiency. Human health effects include: 1) Infection, 2) allergy, 3) irritation, and 4) toxicity.

Infection

Most fungi use non-living material (saprophytes) but a few are pathogens and will invade human tissue. Some saprobes can also cause infection and impact the health of building occupants. Fungi that cause human disease often exist in both mycelial and a unicellular yeast form. These are called "dimorphic" fungi. The conversion is often related to temperature. At room temperature, the fungi are mycelial; at body temperature, they are yeast-like (Rippon, 1998). Four general types of infectious disease are caused by fungi: 1) **cutaneous infections**; 2) **subcutaneous mycosis**; 3) **systemic mycosis**, where fungus is disseminated throughout the body in an otherwise normal host, and 4) **opportunistic infections,** where the fungus invades human tissues, when the host defenses are impaired.

Allergy

A wide range of fungal species are related to antigenic and allergenic disease. It is thought that all mould species are potentially allergenic given adequate exposure, but *Alternaria, Auerobasidium, Cladosporium, Chaetomium,* etc. are known allergenic species. Although wood decay fungi are not normally associated with indoor air quality, their spores are some of the most potent of the fungal allergens. Antigens are substances that induce an immune response. An antigen is called an allergen when it stimulates production of immunoglobulin antibodies. Fungi produce a variety of compounds that are potentially antigenic and allergenic. Sensitization normally occurs through airborne exposure. Two types caused by airborne fungal antigens are allergic diseases (asthma and rhinitis) and hypersensitivity pneumonitis.

Irritation

Fungi produce metabolites and secondary metabolites, depending on conditions and the substrate being digested. Some of these are given off in gaseous form, as volatile organic compounds. Even toxic gas can be released, depending on the species and substrate on which it grows. For example, a fungus growing on wallpaper releases the highly toxic gas arsine, from arsenic containing pigments (Gravesen et. al. 1994). VOCs result in moldy odors and may cause irritation of the mucous membrane of eyes and respiratory system. Fungal volatile compounds (VOCs) may also impact a "common chemical sense" which responds to pungency. Higher level of VOCs exposure from any source and mucous membrane irritants and can affect the central nervous system, resulting in headache, attention deficit, inability to concentrate or dizziness (Amman, 2000).

Toxicity

Many moulds produce mycotoxins and antibiotics, which are secondary metabolites. It is thought that these poisons are produced to provide a competitive advantage over other fungi and bacteria to limit the growth of competing colonies, or to kill them so that they can be digested and consumed. Though intended to damage competing microbes, these metabolites are also toxic to the cells of higher plants and animals, including humans. Toxigenic molds vary in their mycotoxin production depending on the substrate on which they grow (Jarvis, 1990). Almost all mycotoxins have an immunosuppressive effect and increase susceptibility to infectious disease. Molds which produce toxins pose excess health risk compared to other molds though the level of exposure to toxic molds that will result in disease is also not yet clearly understood (Miller, 1998).

Toxigenic fungi found in moisture damaged buildings are most commonly *Penicillium*, *Aspergillus* and *Stachybotrys* species. The toxic metabolites from *Penicillium* include nephrotoxic citrinin (produced by *P. citrinum*, *P. expansum* and *P. viridicatum*), nephrotoxic ochratoxin from *P. cyclopium* and *P. viridicatum*). Toxins from *Aspergillus* species include aflatoxins produced by *A. paraciticus* and *A. flavus*, sterigatocystin from *A. versicolor*, and tremorgenic toxins in the conidia of *A. fumigatus* (Smith and Moss, 1985). Aflatoxin exposure has been linked to liver cancer. *Stachybotrys chartarum* (atra) produces macrocyclic tricothecenes, which have been attributed to causing health symptoms including headache, sore throat, hairs loss, flu symptoms, diarrhea, fatigue, dermatitis, general malaise, and psychological depression (Croff et al. 1986; Jarvis, 1995). Many other species which grow in buildings can produce a variety of other toxins though their occurrence may be less common, including those from *Alternaria*, *Epicoccum*, *Fusarium*, *Trichoderma*, and a few *Cladosporium*.

CONCLUSION

Biodeterioration implies a change in the value of the material which makes the material less useful in aesthetic or utilitarian terms. During the service life of buildings, natural aging and eventual damage of materials due to different chemical, physical and biological processes can take place. Ageing of the materials is one aspect of the environmental processes and involve different chemical, mechanical and biological reactions of the materials biodeterioration, e.g. mould, decay and insect damage in buildings is caused, when moisture exceeds the tolerance of the structures which may be a critical factor for durability and usage of different building materials.

Fungi will grow on damp/moist biodegradable construction and finishing materials. The primary environmental factor controlling the growth of fungi in buildings is moisture availability. Moisture can enter buildings from sources such as rainwater as pipe/sprinkler leaks. Moisture can also occur in building materials from less obvious sources involving water vapor migration and infiltration of humid outdoor air into the building envelope. The typical mould fungi in water damaged finishing building are Ascomycetes fungi: *Alternaria, Penicillium, Fusarium, Aspergillus, Trichoderma, Acremonium* species. Mould fungi cause several problems in buildings — stains, and smell, health problems. Three different decay types are classified and found also in buildings — brown rot, soft rot and white rot. Most of the brown rot and white rot fungi belong to *Basidiomycetes*, but some belong to *Ascomycetes*. Many moulds produce mycotoxins and antibiotics, which are secondary metabolites. It is thought that these poisons are produced to provide a competitive advantage over other fungi and bacteria to limit the growth of competing colonies, or to kill them so that they can be digested and consumed. Many other species which grow in buildings can produce a variety of other toxins though their occurrence may be less common, including those from *Alternaria*, *Epicoccum*, *Fusarium*, *Trichoderma*, and a few *Cladosporium*. Hence the majority of environmental problems in buildings are associated with lack of maintenance, chronic neglect and building defects leading to water ingress, condensation and dampness in the building fabric. The causes of deterioration are influenced by the interval building environment which has a varied microclimate depending upon the building structure and the envelope of the internal building fabric. Buildings affect the health of occupants in many ways, e.g. building-related illness (BRI), sick building syndrome (SBS) and allergy and environmental health problems (AEHP). Management of biodeterioration and health problems in buildings in a complex issue required a multidisciplinary integrated approach which combines the skill of material scientist, environmental monitoring and health specialists, conservation science engineers and architects.

REFERENCES

1. Amman HM. 2000. "Is Indoor Mold Contamination a Threat to Health", Web Page by the Washington state Department of Health, Olympia, Washington.

2. ACGIH 1999 Bioaerosols Assessment and Control. American Confrence of Governmental Industrial Hygienists, Cincinnati, Ohio.

3. Airaksinen M, Jarnstrom H, Kovanen K et al. 2007. Ventilation and building-related symptoms. WellBeing Indoors-CLIMA 2007, 10–14 June, Helsinki.

4. Barnett HL. 2003. Mannual for Hyphomycetes fungi APS publication st. Paul, Minnesota 55121-2097, USA.

5. Burge, H.A. (2000). "The Fungi" In: *Indoor Air Quality Handbook*, Spengler, J.D., Samet, J.M., and McCarthy, J.F.(Editors), McGraw-Hill, New York (U.S.A.), p. 45–1–45.33.

6. Burge, H.A., (1990) *"The Fungi"*, *Biological Contaminants in Indoor Environments*, ASTM STP 1071, Philip R. Morey, James C.Feeley, Sr., James A. Otten, Editors, American Society for Testing and Materials, Philadelphia, 1990. p. 136–162 .

7. Croft , W.A., Jarvis, B.B., Yatawara, C.S. (1986) " Airborne outbreak of trichothecen toxicosis". *Atmos. Environ*, 20(3): 549–552.

8. Chew G.L; Rogers C; Burge H.A; Muilenberg M.L and Gold D.R 2003. Dustborne and airborne fungal propagules and represents a different spectrum of fungi with differing relation to home characteristics. *Allergy*, 58:13–20.

9. Gravesen, S., Frisvad, J.C., Samson, R.A.(1994) " Description of some common fungi". In: *Microfungi*, Munksgaard, Copenhagen, p. 141.

10. Grant, C; Hunter, C.A; Flannigan, B. and Bravery, A.F. 1989. The moisture requriments of moulds isolated from domestic dwellings. *Internat. Biodet*. 25: 259–284.

11. Garner D and Machin K, 2009. Investigation and management of an outbreak of mucormycosis in a paediatric oncology unit. *J Hosp Infect*. 70: 53–59.

12. Hyvarinen A, Meklin T, Vepsalainen A, Nevalainen A, 2002. Fungi and actinobacteria in moisture- damaged building materials- concentrations and diversity. *International Biodeterioration and Biodegradation* 49: 27–37.

13. IOM (2000) Clearing the Air: Asthama and Indoor Air Exposures, Institute of Medicine, National Academy Press, Washington, DC.

14. Jarvis, B.B. (1995) "Mycotoxins in the air: keepour building dry of the bogeyman will get you" Proceeding of the International Conference: Fungi and Bacteria in Indoor Environments. Health Effects, Detection and Remediation EcKardt, J. and Chin S.Y. Saratoga springs, NY, October 6–7, 1994.

15. Jarvis, B.B. (1990) " Mycotoxins and indoor air quality", In: *Biological Contaminants in Indoor Environments*, ASTM Symposium, Boulder, CO, July 16-19, 1989. Morey, P.R., Feeley, J.C., Otten, J.A. eds., p. 201–214.

16. Kumar, M and Verma, R.K. 2010. Fungi diversity and, their effects on building materials, occupants and control-a brief view. *Journal of Scientific and Industrial Research.* 69: 657–661.

17. Leivo, V. and Rantala, J. 2008. Microbiological Aspects of Slab-on–ground Structures. Proceedings of the BEST 1 conferences, Minneapolis, USA, June 12–13.

18. Macher, J., Amman, H.A., Burge, H.A., Milton, D.K., and Morey, P.R. (Editor) (1999) Bioaerosols: Assessment and Control, Cincinnati, OH, American Conference of Governmental Industrial Hygienists.

19. Miller, J.D.,(1998) "Building Related Illness in the Non-Industrial Workplace", Paper Presented to the American Bar Association Meeting, August 4, 1998, Toronto Canada.

20. Morey, P.R., Horner, E., Epstein, B.L., Worthan, A.G., Black, M.S. (2000) "Indoor Air Quality in Nonindustrial Occupational Environments", In: Patly's Industrial Hygiene, Harris, R.L.(Ed.),New York: John Wiely and Sons, V.4

21. Morey, P.R.(1997) "Building Related Illness with a Focus on Fungal Issues", In: A Guide to Managing Indoor Air Quality, Oakbrook Treeace, IL, Joint Commission on Accreditation of Healthcare Organizations.

22. Morey P. Mold growth in building: Removal and Prevention. *Proceeding of Indoor Air* 96, Nagoya, Japan.(1996); Vol. 2: 27–36.

23. Paajanen, L., Ritschkoff, A. and Viitanen, H.(1994). Effect of insulation materials on the biodeterioration of buildings. Espoo. VTT Julkaisuja 791. 64 p. + app. 8p. (Finnish, English Abstract).

24. Ponikau, J.U., Sherris, D.A., Kern, E.B. Homburger, H.A., Frigas, E., Gaffey, T.A. and Roberts, G.D.(1999) "The Diagnosis and Incidence of Allergic Fungal Sinusitis", Mayo Clinic Proceedings, September 1999, Vol 74, p.877–S884.

25. Rippon, J.(1998) *Medical Mycology*, 3d ed. Philadelphia: Saunders.

26. Smith, J.E., Moss, M.O; 1985. *Mycotoxins: Formation, Analysis, and Significance*, John Wiley and Sons, NY.

27. Soikkeli, A.A study on the long-term durability of external wood cladding in Finlnd (2000). In: Soikkeli, A.(ed.). *Management of Europe Building Heritage*. University of Oulu, Department of Architecture. P 100–103.

28. Vitanen, H. (1994).Factor affectingthe development of biodeterioration in wooden construction. *Materials and Structures* 27, 483–493.

29. Viitanen H. 1997a. Modelling the time factor in the development of mould fungi- Effect of critical humidity and temperature conditions in pine and spruce sapwood. *Holzforschung*, vol 51, No1, p. 6–14.

30. Viitanen, H and Salonaara, M. 2001. Failure Criteria. In Trechsel, H.ed. Moisture analysis and Condensation control in building envelopes, MNL 40.ASTM USA. pp. 66–80.

31. Viitanen, H. Hanhijarvi, A. Hukka, A; Koskela, K.(2000). Modelling mould growth and decay damages Health Building 2000: Espoo, 6-10.8 2000. Vol.3.SIY, pp. 341–346.

10

Microbial Biotechnology Moving Towards Nanotechnology

Padma Singh • Deepika Srivastava

INTRODUCTION

Nanotechnology is a new area of science that involves working with materials and devices that are at the nanoscale level. It is the study of matter on an atomic and molecular scale. The nanotechnology was firstly introduced by physicist **Richard Feynman's** speech at the American Physical Society meeting on the topic "**There is plenty of room at the bottom**" at Caltech (US) on December 29, 1959 which emphasis that if our small minds, for some convenience, divide this universe into parts, physics, biology, geology, astronomy, psychology and so on—remember that nature does not know it (Feynman, 1963). He described a process by which the ability to manipulate individual atoms and molecules might be developed and also noted scaling issues would arise from the changing magnitude of various physical phenomena such as gravity would become less important, surface tension and van der Waals attraction would become more significant.

In 1974, Professor Norio Taniguchi of Tokyo Science University defined nanotechnology as "**Nanotechnology mainly consists of the processing, separation, consolidation,** and **deformation of materials by one atom or by one molecule**" (Taniguchi, 1974). In 1980, Dr. Eric Dexler promoted the technological significance of nano-scale phenomena and devices through the speeches and the book "**Engines of creation: The Coming Era of Nanotechnology**" (1986). This book is considered as the first book on the topic of nanotechnology (Drexler, 1991). Further there was invention of scanning tunnelling microscope (STM), carbon nanotubes, and atomic force microscope. In 2000, to coordinate Ferderal nanotechnology research and development, the United States National Nanotechnology (USNN) was founded.

Nanotechnology will be useful in many areas including detection of toxins, pathogens and spoilage in food and food processing facilities, localization and monitoring of diseases in humans, detection of bioterrorism, environmental toxins and assessing effectiveness of remediation processes. It will also have useful application in the fields of nutrition and mutational supplements. Biosensors may detect the presence of chemicals indicating deficiencies of nutrients even before any recognizable symptoms appear and nanomaterials may be used to deliver specific amount of nutrients directly to tissues and cells that needs them. Living cells have been harnessed to produce nanoparticles, such as silver nanoparticles produced extracellularly by the fungus *Aspergillus fumigatus* (Bhainsa and D'Souza, 2006), gold and silver nanoparticles can also be produced by other fungi and a number of bacterial species (Bhattacharya and Gupta, 2005).

According to **21st August 2008**, the **"Project on emerging nanotechnologies"** it is estimated that over 800 manufacturer identified nanotech products are publicly available, some nanoparticles such as titanium dioxide are used in sunscreen, cosmetics and some food products, silver in food packaging, clothing and disinfectants and household appliances, zinc oxide in sunscreen and cosmetics, surface coatings, paints and outdoor furniture varnishes and cerium oxide as fuel catalyst.

NANOTECHNOLOGY IN MICROBIOLOGY

The integration of nanotechnology and microbiology holds tremendous opportunities and can unfold solutions in new ways altering the thinking of scientific realm. Beside the detection of microorganisms and their cellular products such as LPS, enzymes and toxins, nanotechnology and nanomedicines hold great promise for advanced diagnostics and biosensors, targeted drugs delivery and smart drugs, immunoisolation therapies, nanoactuators and nanomotors, microscopic energy sources and nanocomputers at the molecular scale (Fritas, 2002). Biomimetics are now used as an engineering tool, both modeling and reproducing the structure of organism that nature has already developed and refined, creating nanoscale devices, nanomachines and nanoobjects. As nanotechnology develops more methods to manipulate and control matter with fewer molecules, at even smaller sizes, with ever greater precisioness, this will enable microbiologists to refine their research by targeting single receptors, tracking specific molecules, better understanding intracellular signalling cascades, and cellular microbiology which will help to evolve new advantage in nanotechnology.

APPLICATIONS OF NANOTECHNOLOGY

Food Industry

Nanotechnology has been traditionally used in food by food chemist to manipulate food, improving their nutritional value, smart packaging, detecting the presence of pathogens and toxins in food and food processing.

Food Packaging

By using nanocomposite materials, improvements are being made in characteristics of food packaging materials, such as strength, barrier properties, antimicrobial properties and stability to heat and cold. **Polymer**–silicate nanocomposites have also been reported to have improved gas barrier properties, mechanical strength and thermal stability (Holley, 2005; Schaefer, 2005, Brody, 2006). Nanotechnology can also help in detecting food deterioration. Nanoclay—nylon coatings and silicon oxide barriers for glass bottles that impede gas diffusion, metallised films, and antimicrobials incorporated in packaging, smarter bar codes, and improved pigments, inks and adhesives.

Food Processing

There are several food processing methods which use enzymes to alter food components to improve flavour, nutritional value or other characteristics. Immobilization of these enzymes on nanoparticles may aid in dispersion through food matrices and enhance their activity. Nano-silicon dioxide particles with reactive aldehyde groups were made and found to be covalently bound to porcine triacylglcerol lipase. These particles effectively hydrolyzed olive oil and were determined to have good stability, adoptability and reusability (Bai *et al.*, 2006).

Cleaning and Disinfection

In the presence of UV light, titanium dioxide generates reactive species such as hydroxyl and superoxide radicals that cause degradation of organic compounds and bacteria. Deposition of silver on nanoparticles of titanium dioxide increases its bacteriocidal effects against *E. coli* (Kim *et al.*, 2006) while titanium dioxide combined with carbon nanotubes has enhanced disinfectant properties against *Bacillus cereus* spores (Krishna *et al.*, 2005). Silver doped titanium dioxide nanoparticles also inactivated *Bacillus cereus* spores on aluminium and polyester surfaces (Vohra A. *et al.*, 2005) and destroyed air-borne bacteria and molds, when incorporated into an air filter (Vohra *et al.*, 2006). Silver is having antibacterial effects and nanoparticles of silver stabilized with SDS or PVP effectively inhibited growth of *E. coli* and *Staphylococcus aureus* (Cho *et al.*, 2005).

Sensors

Detection of very small amounts of a chemical, virus or bacteria in food system is one of the potential application of nanotechnology. Nanosensors that are being developed can either be tailor made to fluoresce different colours or alternately be manufactured out of magnetic materials. These nanoparticles can then selectively attach themselves to any number of pathogen. The advantage of this system is that hundreds and thousands of nanoparticles can be placed on a single nanosensor to rapidly, accurately and affordably detect the presence of any number of different bacteria and pathogens and the second advantage is that, their small size, due to which they gain access into the tiny crevices where the pathogen often hide. Improved biosensor technology may be used for detecting the gases present in the packaged foods, which may detect the compound released during food spoilage or deterioration and the presence of pathogens or toxins in food.

Numerous recent research paper describe detection methods for bacteria, viruses, toxins or other organic compounds based on nanotechnological methods and devices. Such as – immunosensing of *Staphylococcus enterotoxin* B (SEB) in milk was achieved using polydimethylsiloxane (PDMS) chips with reinforced, supported fluid bilayer membrane. Antibodies to SEB were attached to the bilayer membrane in PDMS channels to form a biosensor with a detection limit of 0.5 ng/ml (Dong *et al.*, 2006).

An immunomagnetic bead sandwich assay using universal G-liposomal nanovesicles in an array-based system was developed to simultaneously detect *E. coli* O157:H7, *Salmonella* spp. and *Listeria monocytogenes*. In mixed cultures, limits of detection were $3.1 \times 10_3$, $7.8 \times 10_4$, $7.9 \times 10_5$, respectively (Chen and Durst, 2006). An electrochemical glucose biosensor, with detection and quantification limits 0.035 and 0.107 mM, respectively, was nanofabricated by layer-by-layer self-assembly of polyelectrolytes on an electrode platform. Multi-walled carbon nanotubes dispersed in the perfluorosulfonated polymer, nafion, were deposited on a glassy carbon electrode followed by absorption of a chitosan derivative as a polycation and glucose oxidase as a biorecognition element. Glucose in solution was detected by changes in current (Rivas *et al.*, 2006). Liposome nanovesicles have been devised to detect peanut allergenic proteins in chocolate (Wen *et al.*, 2005) and pathogens (Edwards and Baeumner, 2006).

Medicine

Nanoscience and nanotechnology are spurring the development of more sophisticated tools for detecting diseases such as cancer and atherosclerosis at early stages, delivering drugs to specific sites in the bodies and performing neurosurgery. Novel nanostructures can serve as new kinds of drugs for treating common condition such as cancer, Parkinson's and cardiovascular disease, or as artificial tissues for replacing diseased kidneys and liver.

Applications of nanotechnology in diagnosis of disease are developing rapidly. Two targets associated with atherosclerosis, fibrin and tissue factor, can be detected by MRI using paramagnetic nanoparticles targeted to these proteins and by use of targeted echogenic liposomes that alternate lipid bilayers with an aqueous fluid and produce an ultrasound signal (Wickline *et al.*, 2006). Nanoparticles of superparamagnetic iron oxide can also be used to visualize brain tumors using MRI (Muldoon *et al.*, 2006). Specific nanoparticles can also be combined with nanowires, nanotubes, nanocantilevers, and microarrays to produce integrated and automated detection systems (Leary *et al.*, 2006).

Nanoparticles may also aid in delivering drugs directly to tissue targets. Among applications under development are:

a. Nanoparticles specific for smooth muscle cells that are loaded with paclitaxel or fumigallin that inhibit plaque development on artery walls (Wickline *et al.*, 2006) and poly(lactide)-tocopheryl polyethylene glycol succinate particles to efficiently deliver the cancer drug, paclitaxel (Zhang and Feng, 2006);

b. "Stealth" nanoparticles that circumvent the bloodbrain barrier and deliver drugs to attack brain tumors (Muldoon *et al.*, 2006);

c. RNA nanoparticles containing siRNA (small interfering RNA) and folate for treatment of nasopharyngeal carcinoma.

These nanoparticles would bind to the membranes and bring the siRNA into the cells (Guo *et al.*, 2006). Restorative materials that aid in healing or replace damaged body parts may also be improved by nanotechnology. Nanoparticles of quaternary ammonium polyethylimine have been incorporated in composite resins used in dentistry to replace hard tissues. Such resins exerted antibacterial effects against *Streptococcus mutans* for at least one month and did not diminish the structural integrity of the resin (Beyth *et al.*, 2006). Nanocrystals of hydroxyapatite-aspartic acid (or-glutamic acid) have been found to interact with osteoblasts and enhance their activity in mineralization reactions. These composites may be useful in treatment of osteoporosis and other bone diseases (Boanini *et al.*, 2006). Nanofibers of a peptide amphiphile have been used to construct a scaffold that attached mesenchymal stem cells and enhanced their proliferation and differentiation. This system may also be useful for tissue repair (Boanini *et al.*, 2006). In a procedure called "nano-neuro-knitting," one research group described the use of **SAPNS** (self-assembling peptide nanofiber scaffolds) to repair a severed optic nerve tract in hamsters. Regeneration of axons (elongated parts of nerve cells) after traumatic injury or a stroke is very difficult because of the formation of scar tissue, gaps in nervous tissue caused by phagocytosis of damaged cells, and the inability of many adult neurons to initiate axonal growth. **SAPNS** are self-assembling peptides with alternating positive and negative L-amino acids that form interwoven nanofibers (about 10 nm in diameter) that form a highly hydrated scaffolds in human body fluids, culture media, and even saline solutions. This scaffolding bridges the damaged tissue providing a framework for the partial regrowth and connection of nerve cells. Approximately 80% of nerves were regenerated in both adult and young animals in the best cases and some regrowth was evident after only 24 hours (Ellis-Behnke *et al.*, 2006).

Biomedical Sciences

This technology plays a vital role in various biomedical applications such as:

- Tissue engineering (Ma *et al.*, 2003; de la Isla *et al.*, 2003)
- Drug and gene delivery (Mah *et al.*, 2000; Panatarotto *et al.*, 2003)
- Detection of proteins (Nam *et al.*, 2000)
- Biodetection of pathogens (Edelstein *et al.*, 2000)
- Probing of DNA structures (Mahtab *et al.*, 1995)
- Tumor destruction by heating (hyperthermia) (Yoshida and Kobayashi, 1999)
- MRI contrast enhancement (Weissleder *et al.*, 1990)
- Separation and purification of biomolecules and cells (Molday and Mackenzie, 1982)
- Fluorescent biological markers (Bruchez *et al.*, 1998; Chan and Nie, 1998)
- Artificial cells and their assemblies (Pohorille and Deamer, 2002)
- Design of proteins for efficient electron or with mechanical features (Gilardi *et al.*, 2002)
- Using dip pen technology (Hyun *et al.*, 2002; Liu and Amro, 2002)
- Formation and growth of nanostructures in living biosystem (e.g by alfalfa plant) (Gardea-Torresdey *et al.*, 2002)
- Biosensors (Tiefenauer and Ros, 2002)
- Nanobiomotors (Moore and Prevelige, 2002; Liu *et al.*, 2002; Roco, 2001)
- Biomineralization (Banfield and Navrosky, 2002)
- Nanorobotics (Freitas, 1999; Drexler, 1992)
- Nanocomputers (Collier *et al.*, 2000)
- Nanorods for vaccination applications (Salem *et al.*, 2005)

Nanotechnology has a prominent use in target specific drug therapy and methods for early diagnosis of pathologies. The National Institutes of Health Bioengineering Consortium (BECON) held a symposium in 2000 entitled "**Nanoscience and Technology: Shaping Biomedical Research**" (BECON Nanoscience and Nanotechnology Symposium Report, 2005), in which, eight areas where believed to be the most pertinent to research in biomedicine. These include synthesis and use of nanostructure, applications of nanotechnology to therapy, biomimetic and biologic nanostructure, electronic-biology interface, devices for early detection of disease, tools for the study of single molecules, nanotechnology and tissue engineering.

Most important clinical application of nanotechnology is in pharmaceutical development. These applications take advantage of the unique properties of nanoparticles as drugs or constituent of drugs or are designed for new strategies to controlled release, drug targeting, and salvage of drugs with low bioavailability (Roy et al., 2003; Brigger et al., 2002; Crommelin et al., 2003).

Nanoscale polymer capsules can be designed to breakdown and release drugs at controlled rates, to allow differential release in certain environments, such as an acid medium, and to promote uptake in tumours versus normal tissues (Na and Bae, 2002). Nanocapsules can be synthesized directly from monomers or by means of nanodeposition of preformed polymers (Couvreur et al., 2002). Nanocapsules have also been formulated from albumin and liposomes. Implantable drug delivery systems are also being developed which will make use of nanopores to control drug release.

Despite the risk and limitations, viral vectors are an efficient biomimetic approach to drug targeting and delivery. The tat peptide from human immunodeficiency virus (HIV) and other viral proteins are being attacked to DNA, proteins and other materials for uptake into cells. These nano-assemblies mimic the action of the fusion proteins that make viral transfection efficient (Lewin et al., 2000; Reynolds et al., 2003).

By the help of nanotechnology, there can be exploration in the research of repair of the brain and other areas for regaining cognition. It can also help in the production of implantable detectors with minimal quantity of blood. It should also be possible to develop methods that used saliva instead of blood for the detection of illnesses or that can perform complete blood testing within a short period of time.

Nanodevices in medical sciences can be used to replace defective or improperly functioning cells, such as the respirocyte proposed by Freitas (Freitas, 1996). This man-made red blood cell is theoretically capable of providing oxygen more effectively than an erythrocyte. It could replace defective natural red cells in blood circulation. Primary application of respirocytes may involve transfusable blood substitution, partial treatment of anaemia, prenatal/neonatal problems, and lung disorders.

Nanorobots are also one of the applications of nanotechnology. Nanorobots operating in the human body, could monitor levels of different compounds and record the information in the internal memory. They could be rapidly used in the examination of a given tissue, surveying its biochemical, biomechanical, and histometrical features in detail. Nanoparticulate carriers have been developed as on solution to overcome such delivery problems, i.e. drugnanocrystals, solid lipid nanoparticles (SLN) nanostructured lipid carriers (NLC) and lipid-drug conjugate (LDC) nanoparticles (Muller and Keck, 2004). The carriers as reported by Muller and colleagues are suitable to solve delivery problems with biotech drugs of different solubility. Targeting with these carriers can be realised by a very simple approach, the differential proteins adsorption (path finder technology). This technology proved to be efficient enough to accumulate sufficiently high amount of drugs in the brain to reach therapeutic levels and also fulfil the major requirement to be pursued by a pharmaceutical company.

Quantum Dot could offer a cheap and easy way to screen a blood sample for the presence of a number of different viruses and at the same time, it could also give physician a fast diagnosis tool to detect, say, the presence of a particular set of proteins that strongly indicates the onset of myocardial infarction (Quantum Dot Corporation, 2005).

The RESIST Group at the Welsh School of Pharmacy at Cardiff University and others have looked at how molecularly imprinted polymers could be medically useful in clinical applications such as controlled drug release, drug monitoring devices, and biological and antibody receptor mimics. Histamine and ephedrine molecularly imprinted polymers (MIPs) were studied as potential biological receptor mimics whilst a propanolol MIP was investigated for its use as a rate attenuating selective excipient in a transdermal controlled device (Allender *et al.*, 2000).

The first artificial voltage-gated molecular **nanosieve** was fabricated by Charles R. Martin and colleagues (Nishizawa *et al.*, 1995) at Colorado State University in 1995. Martin's membrane contains an array of cylindrical gold nanotubules with inside diameters as small as 1.6 nm nanofibers as nanosieve. When the tubules are positively charged, positive ions are excluded and only negative ions are transported through the membrane. When the membrane receives a negative voltage, only positive ions can pass. Similar nanodevices may combine voltage gating with pore size, shape, and charge constraints to achieve precise control of ion transport with significant molecular specificity. An exquisitely sensitive ion channel switch biosensor was built by an Australian research group (Cornell *et al.*, 1997).

Calcium phosphate nanoparticles present a unique class of non-viral vectors, which can serve as efficient and alternative DNA carriers for targeted delivery of genes. The design and synthesis of ultra-low size, highly monodispersed DNA doped calcium phosphate nanoparticles of size around 80 nm in diameter has been reported (Roy *et al.*, 2003). The DNA encapsulated inside the nanoparticle is protected from the external DNase environment and could be used safely to transfer the encapsulated DNA under *in vitro* and *in vivo* conditions.

The application of a combination of nanomedicine with biophotonics for optically tracking the cellular pathways of gene delivery and the resulting transfection by using nanoparticles as a non-viral vector has been demonstrated recently (Roy *et al.*, 2005). Gene delivery is an area of considerable current interest; genetic materials (DNA, RNA, and oligonucleotides) have been used as molecular medicine and are delivered to specific cell types to either inhibit some undesirable gene expression or express therapeutic proteins.

Nanoparticles as Biomarker

Nanoparticles can be used for both quantitative and qualitative *in vitro* detection of tumour cells. They enhance the detection process by concentrating and protecting a marker from degradation, in order to render the analysis more sensitive. For instance, streptavidin-coated fluorescent polystyrene nanospheres Fluospheres® (green fluorescence) and TransFluospheres® (red fluorescence) were applied in single colour flow cytometry to detect the epidermal growth factor receptor (EGFR) on A 431 cells (human epidermoid carcinoma cells) (Bhalgat *et al.*, 1998). The results have shown that the fluorescent nanospheres provided a sensitivity of 25 times more than that of the conjugate streptavidin-fluorescein.

Contrast agents have been loaded on to nanoparticles for tumour diagnosis purposes. The physico-chemical features (particle size, surface charge, surface coating, and stability) of the nanoparticles allow the redirection and the concentration of the marker at the specific site of interest. Labelled colloidal particles could be used as radiodiagnostic agents. On the other hand, some non-labelled colloidal systems are already in use and some are still being tested as contrast agents in related diagnosis procedures such as computed tomography and NMR imaging.

To date, a study of radionuclide use in diagnostic imaging with nanoparticles for cancer detection is yet to be published. However, as conventional colloidal particles can be cells of organs like the liver, the spleen, the lungs and the bone marrow and as long-circulating nanoparticles can have a compartmental localization in the blood circulation or the lymphatic system — all these organs being potential sites for tumour development, these colloidal systems could potentially improve tumour diagnosis.

In the future, nanoparticles that are engineered with specific binding affinities can be resuspended into the collected body fluids, or perhaps even injected directly into the circulation. The nanoparticles, together with the bound molecules, could be directly captured on engineered filters and directly questioned by ultra-high-resolution mass spectrometry, e.g. Fourier Transform Ion Cyclotron Resonance.

Measurements of Dissolved Oxygen

Oxygen is one of the major metabolites in aerobic systems, and the measurement of dissolved oxygen is of vital importance in medical, industrial, and environmental applications. Recent interest in the methods for measuring dissolved oxygen concentration has been focused mainly on optical sensors, due to their advantages over conventional amperometric electrodes in that they are faster, do not consume oxygen, and are not easily poisoned (Xu *et al.*, 2001; McDonagh *et al.*, 1998).

Optical **PEBBLE (probes encapsulated by biologically localized embedding)** nanosensors have been developed for dissolved oxygen using organically modified silicate (ormosil) nanoparticles as a matrix. The ormosil nanoparticles are prepared through a sol-gel-based process, which includes the formation of core particles with phenyltrimethoxysilane as a precursor followed by the formation of a coating layer with methyltrimethoxysilane as a precursor (Koo Lee *et al.* 2004). The highly permeable structure and the hydrophobic nature of the ormosil nanoparticles, as well as their small size, result in an excellent overall quenching response to dissolved oxygen and a linear response over the whole range, from 0–100% oxygen-saturated water. This PEBBLE sensor has a higher sensitivity and a broader linearity as well as longer excitation and emission wavelengths, resulting in reduced background noise for cellular measurement. The PEBBLE sensors are excellent in terms of their reversibility and stability to leaching and long-term storage. A real-time monitoring of changes in the dissolved oxygen due to cell respiration in a closed chamber was made by gene gun delivered PEBBLE. This sensor is now being applied for simultaneous intracellular measurements of oxygen and glucose (Koo Lee *et al.*, 2004).

Use of Nanotechnology to P450 Enzymes

Cytochromes P450 are highly relevant to the bio-analytical area (Sadeghi *et al.*, 2001). They form a large family of enzymes present in all tissues essential to the metabolism of most drugs in use today, playing a vital role in the drug development and discovery process. They act as catalysts for the insertion of one of the two atoms of an oxygen molecule into a variety of substrates (R) with quite broad regioselectivity, leading to concomitant reduction of the other oxygen atom to water (Gilardi *et al.*, 2002).

$$RH + O_2 + 2e^- + 2H^+ \rightarrow ROH + H_2O$$

Several methods have been reported in the literature for the screening of substrate turnover by P450s in a high throughput format (Joo *et al.*, 1999; Dmochowski *et al.*, 1999; Grigoryev *et al.*, 1999; Schwaneberg *et al.*, 1999). However, they all fall short of being limited to testing the activity of P450 enzymes through the detection of the conversion of a specific marker substrate, but (Tsotsou *et al.* 2002) have been able to develop a method called the alkali method, which can detect the turnover of any NAD (P) H or NAD (P) + dependent enzyme. The progress on these research fronts and their combinations provide a powerful platform for future applications of these enzymes, with particular reference to protein array technology.

Tissue Engineering

Tissue engineering is based on the creation of new tissues *in vitro* followed by surgical placement in the body or the stimulation of normal repair in situ using bioartificial constructs or implants of living cells introduced in or near the area of damage. Though it is mainly concerned with using human material, either from the patients themselves (autologous) or from other human sources **(allogeneic)**, material from other mammalian sources has also been applied in humans **(xenogeneic)**. The involvement of microelectronics or nanotechnology in creating a truly bioartificial tissue or organ that can take the place of one that is terminally diseased, such as an eye, ear, heart, or joint has been envisaged. Implantable prosthetic devices and nanoscaffolds for use in the growing of artificial organs are goals of nanotechnology researchers. Nanoengineering of hydroxyapatite for bone replacement is reasonably advanced (Wang *et al.*, 2002; Du *et al.*, 1998). In the future, we could imagine a world where medical nanodevices are routinely implanted or even injected into the bloodstream to monitor wellness and to automatically participate in the repair of systems that deviate from established norms. These nanobots could be personalized by tailoring them to patient genotype and phenotype to optimize intervention at the earliest stage in the course of disease expression (Thrall, 2004).

Growth of New Organs (Fig. 10.1)

Nanoscale building of cells can be accomplished by their programmed replication. The signals are transmitted back and forth with the instruction for the desired size and shape form the construction site. When complete instructions are finished, the organs can be grown according to the prerequisite specifications. These organs could have the necessary DNA encoded to be compatible with the required human body immunological status. This can enhance integration of artificial structures with living tissues, presenting a more appropriate interface to biological systems. With the advantage in absence of immune reaction unlike today's donor organ transplantation. In the years to come, this, can accomplish a quantum leap in the management of organ failure disorders.

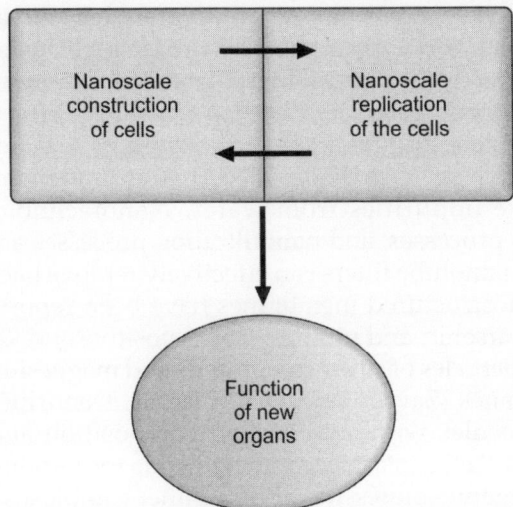

Fig. 10.1: Nanoscale construction and growth of new organs

Molecular Imaging

New imaging approaches using genetically encoded fluorescent and bioluminescent reporters (i.e. illuminated or glowing identification tags) are offering revealing insights to the living body as never observed before. Information provided by these reporters can be used to enhance our understanding of human biology and the development of therapeutic approaches for many diseases, including cancer, infection, neurodegenerative and cardiovascular disease.

Pollution Abatement

Provision of sufficient clean water for human consumption, agriculture, and industrial processes is an ongoing and increasing challenge as a result of population growth, extended droughts, and numerous competing demands. Nanotechnology offers several possible novel, improved and efficient methods for purifying water. Photocatalytic membranes have been produced and tested in a pilot plant for their efficacy in degrading triazine herbicides. Use of these compounds particularly in areas with sandy soils has contaminated underground aquifers with compounds such as atrazine. Composite membranes produced by nanotechnology and containing titanium dioxide, tributyl- and triisopropyl vanadate were exposed to sunlight resulting in the oxidation and destruction of atrazine in water at a concentration of 1 ppm (Bellobono *et al.*, 2005). Other systems containing titanium dioxide nanoparticles have been reported to degrade PCBs and other organic pollutants in water (Savage and Diallo, 2006). Nanomaterials can also be used to adsorb or sequester pollutants and remove them from water. Sorbents are already widely used in water purification but nanosorbents can be much more effective because they have a much larger surface area as compared to conventional bulk particles. Various chemical groups can also be added to nanoparticles to improve their specificity in removing certain pollutants. Multiwalled carbon nanotubes have been found to adsorb 3–4 times the amount of heavy metals (copper, cadmium, and lead) as powdered or granular activated carbon. Chitosan nanoparticles containing tripolyphosphate adsorb even greater amounts of lead. Other nanosorbents have been devised to remove arsenic and chromium from water. Carbon nanotubes and nanoporous activated carbon fibers can effectively adsorb organic pollutants such as benzene and fullerenes can adsorb polycyclic aromatic compounds such as naphthalene (Savage and Diallo, 2006). Ultrafiltration and reverse osmosis are now used to remove impurities from water. Nanotechnology can enhance the effectiveness of these processes, and nanofiltration processes are being developed for desalination. Carbon nanotube filters can effectively remove bacteria and viruses from water, and other nanostructured membranes have been reported to remove organic pollutants, uranium, arsenic, and nitrates. Gram-positive and Gram-negative bacteria can be killed by nanoparticles of silver compounds and magnesium oxide which disrupt bacterial cell membranes (Savage and Diallo, 2006). Dendritic polymers are highly branched macromolecules with a controlled composition and architecture. These polymers (1–20 nm in size) can act as soluble ligands for radionuclides, heavy metals, inorganic ions, and organic solutes. Metal-dendrimer complexes can be separated from the solution and the metals released by altering the pH. This would allow reuse of the polymers and recovery of the metals. Dendritic polymers can also act as scaffolds to carry antimicrobial compounds (Savage and Diallo, 2006).

CONCLUSION AND FUTURE PROSPECTS

Till now, nanotechnology is in its infancy. It will affect virtually all of the devices and materials we deal with in everyday life, from consumer products to food to medicine. Even though current application of nanotechnology might seem rather crude, they are advancing. Future applications will become increasingly sophisticated, giving scientists and engineers the ability to tackle challenging problems that affect us all—including treating cancer, generating clean and renewable energy, and providing clean water anytime, anyplace. These new applications will raise important questions concerning how we develop safe and acceptable nanotechnologies. Perhaps the greatest challenge to benefiting from nanotechnology is having the foresight to develop and use it wisely. Drexler concluded Nanosystem as "Each step will present great practical challenges, but each step will also bring valuable new capabilities. This long-term reward, measured in terms of scientific and technological capabilities, appears large."

REFERENCES

1. Allender CJ, Richardson C, Woodhouse B, et al. 2000. "Pharmaceutical applications for molecularly imprinted polymers", *Int. J. Pharm.* 195, 39–43.

2. Bai YX, Li YF, Yang Y, et al. 2006. "Covalent immobilization of triacylglycerol lipase on to functionalized nanoscale SiO_2 spheres". *Process Biochem* 41:770–777.

3. Banfield JF, Navrosky A. 2002. "Nanoparticles and the environment" *Rev. Mineralogy Geochemistry*, 44, 6–16.

4. BECON Nanoscience and Nanotechnology Symposium Report, June (2000). National Institutes of Health Bioengineering Consortium, 2000. National Institute of Health web site, accessed March 20th, 2005.

5. Bellobono IR, Morazzoni F, Bianchi R, et al. 2005. "Photosynthetic membranes, Part 74: Solar energy driven photocatalytic membrane modules for water reuse in agricultural and food industries. Pre-industrial experience using s-triazines as model molecules". *Int J Photoenergy* 7:87–94.

6. Beyth N., Yudovin–Farber I., Bahir R., Domb A.J., and Weissa E. 2006. "Antibacterial activity of dental composites containing quaternary ammonium polyethylenimine nanoparticles against *Streptococcus mutans*". *Biomaterials* 27:3995–4002.

7. Bhainsa K.C. and D'Souza S.F. 2006. "Extracellular biosynthesis of silver nanoparticles using the fungus *Aspergillus fumigatus*". Colloids Surfaces B: *Biointerfaces* 47:160–164.

8. Bhalgat M.K., Haugland R.P., Pollack J.S. and Swan S. 1998. "Green- and Red-Fluorescent Nanospheres for The Detection of Cell Surface Receptors by Flow Cytometry", *J. Immunol. Methods*, 219, 57–68.

9. Bhattacharya D. and Gupta R.K. 2005. "Nanotechnology and potential microorganisms". *Crit Rev Biotechnol* 25:199–20.

10. Boanini E., Torricelli P., Gazzano M., Giardino R., and Bigi A. 2006. "Nanocomposites of hydroxyapatite with aspartic acid and glutamic acid and their interaction with osteoblast-like cells". *Biomaterials* 27:4428–4433.

11. Brigger I., Dubernet C., and Couvreur P. 2002. "Nanoparticles in Cancer Therapy and Diagnosis", *Adv. Drug Deliv. Rev.*, 54,631–651.

12. Brody A.L. 2006. "Nano and food packaging technologies converge". *Food Technol* 60:92–94.

13. Bruchez M., Moronne M., Gin P., Weiss S. and Alivisatos A.P. 1998. "Semiconductor Nanocrystals As Fluorescent Biological Labels". *Science*, 281, 2013–2016.

14. Chan W.C.W. and Nie S.M. 1998. "Quantum Dot Bioconjugates For Ultrasensitive Nonisotopic Detection". *Science*, 281 , 2016–2018.

15. Chen C.S. and Durst R.A. 2006. "Simultaneous detection of *Escherichia coli* O157:H7, *Salmonella spp.* and *Listeria monocytogenes* with an array-based immunosorbent assay using universal protein Gliposomal nanovesicles". *Talanta* 69:232–238.

16. Cho K.H., Park J.E., Osaka T., and Park S.G. 2005. "The study of antimicrobial activity and preservative effects of nanosilver ingredient". *Electrochim Acta* 51:956–960.

17. Collier C.P., Mattersteig G., Wong E.W., Luo Y., Beverly K., Sampaio J., Raymo F.M., Stoddart J.F. and Heath J.R. 2000. "A (2) Catenane-Based Solid State Electronically Reconfigurable Switch". *Science*, 289, 1172–1175.

18. Cornell B., Braach-Maksvytis V., King L., Osman P., Raguse B., Wieczorek L. and Pace R. 1997. "A Biosensor that Uses Ion-Channel Switches". *Nature*, 387, 580–583.

19. Couvreur P., Barratt G., Fattal E., Legrand P. and Vauthier C. 2002. "Nanocapsule Technology: A Review". *Crit. Rev. Ther. Drug. Carrier Syst.*, 19, 99–134.

20. Crommelin D.J., Storm G., Jiskoot W., Stenekes R., Mastrobattista E. and Hennink W.E. 2003. "Nanotechnological Approaches for The Delivery of Macromolecules". *J. Control Release*, 87, 81–88.

21. De la Isla A., Brostow W., Bujard B., Estevez M., Rodriguez J.R., Vagas S. and Castano V.M. 2003. "Nanohybrid Scratch Resistant Coating for Teeth and Bone Viscoelasticity Manifested in Tribology", *Mat. Resr. Innovat.*, 7, 110–114.

22. Dmochowski I.J., Crane B.R., Wilker J.J., Winkler J.R. and Gray H.B.1999. "Optical Detection of Cytochrome P450 by Sensitizer-Linked Substrates". *Proc. Natl. Acad. Sci. USA*, 96, 12987–12990.

23. Dong Y., Phillips K.S., and Chenk Q. 2006. "Immunosensing of Staphylococcus enterotoxin B (SEB) in milk with PDMS microfluidic systems using reinforced supported bilayer membranes (r-SBMs)". *Lab on a Chip* 6:675–681.

24. Drexler E.K. 1992. "Nanosytems: Molecular Machinery, Manufacturing and Computation", John Wiley and Sons, New York.

25. Du C., Cui F.Z., Feng Q.L., Zhu X.D. and de Groot K.1998. "Tissue Response to Nano-Hydroxyapatite/Collagen Composite Implants in Marrow Cavity". *J. Biomed. Mater. Res.*, 42, 540–548.

26. Edelstein R.L., Tamanaha C.R., Sheehan P.E., Miller M.M., Baselt D.R., Whitman L.J. and Colton R.J. 2000. "The Barc Biosensor Applied to The Detection of Biological Warfare Agents". *Biosensors Bioelectron.* 14, 805–813.

27. Edwards K.A. and Baeumner A.J. 2006. "Liposomes in analyses". Talanta 68:1421–1431.

28. Ellis-Behnke R.G., Liang Y.X., You S.W., Tay D.K.C., Zhang S.G., So K.F., and Schneider G.E. 2006. "Nano neuro knitting: Peptide nanofiber scaffold for brain repair and axon regeneration with functional return of vision". *Proc Natl Acad Sci USA* 103:5054–5059.

29. Eric Drexler. 1991. *"Nanosystems: Molecular Machinery, Manufacturing, and Computation. MIT PhD thesis"*. New York: Wiley.

30. Freitas R.A. 1996 "The Future of Computers". *Analog.*, 116, 57–73.

31. Fritas R.A. Jr. 2002. "The future of nanofabrication and molecular scale devices in nanomedicine". *Study of Health Technology Information*; 80:45–59.

32. Gardea-Torresdey J.L., Parsons J.G., Gomez E., Peralta-Videa J., Troiani H.E., Santiago P., and Yacaman M.J. 2002. "Formation And Growth of Au Nanoparticles Inside Alfalfa Plants". *Nano. Lett.*, 2, 397–401.

33. Gilardi G., Meharenna Y. T., Tsotsou G.E., Sadeghi S.J., Fairhead M. and Giannini S. 2002. "Molecular Lego: Design of Molecular Assemblies of P450 Enzymes for Nanobiotechnology". *Biosensors and Bioelectronics*, 17, 133–145.

34. Grigoryev D.N., Kato K., Njar V.C.O., Long B.J., Ling Y.Z., Wang X., Mohler J. and Brodie A.M.H. 1999. "Cytochrome P450c17-Expressing *E. coli* as a First Step Screening System for 17 Alpha-Hydroxylase C17, 20-Lyase Inhibitors". *Anal. Biochem.*, 267, 319–330.

35. Guo S., Huang F., and Guo P. 2006. "Construction of folate-conjugated pRNA of bacteriophage phi29 DNA packaging motor for delivery of chimeric siRNA to nasopharyngeal carcinoma cells". *Gene Therapy* 13:814–820.

36. Holley C. 2005. "Nanotechnology and packaging. Secure protection for the future". *Verpackungs- Rundschau* 56:53–56.

37. Hyun J., Ahn S.J., Lee W.K., Chilkoti A. and Zauscher S. 2002. "Molecular Recognition-Mediated Fabrication of Protein Nanostructures by Dip-Pen Lithography". *Nano. Lett.*, 2, 1203–1207.

38. Joo H., Lin Z. and Arnold F.H. 1999. "Laboratory Evolution of Peroxide-Mediated Cytochrome P450 Hydroxylation". *Nature*, 399, 670–673.

39. Kim K.D., Han D.N., Lee J.B., and Kim H.T. 2006. "Formation and characterization of Ag-deposited TiO_2 nanoparticles by chemical reduction method". *Scripta Materials* 54:143–146.

40. Koo Lee Y.E., Cao Y., Kopelman R., Koo S.M., Brasuel M. and Philbert M.A. 2004. "Real-Time Measurements of Dissolved Oxygen Inside Live Cells by Organically Modified Silicate Fluorescent Nanosensors". *Anal. Chem.*, 76, 2498–2505.

41. Krishna V., Pumprueg S., Lee S.H., Zhao J., Sigmund W., Koopman B., and Moudgil B.M. 2005. "Photocatalytic disinfection with titanium dioxide coated multi-wall carbon nanotubes". *Process Safety Environ Protect* 83:393–397.

42. Leary S.P., Liu C.Y., and Apuzzo M.L.J. 2006. "Toward the emergence of nanoneurosurgery. Part II: Nanomedicine: Diagnostics and imaging at the nanoscale level". *Neurosurgery* 58:805–822.

43. Lewin M., Carlesso N., Tung C. H., et al. 2000. "Tat Peptide-Derivatized Magnetic Nanoparticles Allow in Vivo Tracking and Recovery of Progenitor Cells". *Nat. Biotechnol.*, 18, 410–413.

44. Liu G. and Amro N. 2002. "Positioning Protein Molecules on Surfaces: A Nanoengineering Approach to Supramolecular Chemistry", *Proc. Natl. Acad. Sci.* USA, 99, 5165–5170.

45. Liu H., Schmidt J.J., Bachand G.D., Rizk S.S., Looger L.L., Hellinga H.W. and Montemagno C.D. 2002. "Control of A Biomolecular Motor Powered Nanodevices with an Engineered Chemical Switch". *Nat. Mater.*, 1, 173–177.

46. Ma J., Wong H., Kong L.B. and Peng K.W. 2003. "Biomimetic Processing of Nanocrystalline Bioactive Apatite Coating on Titanium". *Nanotechnology*, 14, 619–623.

47. Mah C., Zolotukhin I., Fraites T.J., Dobson J., Batich C. and Byrne B.J. 2000. "Microsphere-Mediated Delivery of Recombinant AAV Vectors *In-vitro* and *In-vivo*". *Mol. Therapy*, I, S239.

48. Mahtab R., Rogers J.P. and Murphy C.J. 1995. "Protein-Sized Quantum Dot Luminescence can Distinguish Between 'Straight', 'Bent' and 'Kinked' Oligonucleotides", *J. Am. Chem. Soc.*, 117, 9099–9100.

49. McDonagh C., MacCraith B.D. and McEvoy A.K.1998. "Tailoring of Sol-Gel Films for Optical Sensing of Oxygen in Gas and Aqueous Phase". *Anal. Chem.*, 70, 45–50.

50. Molday R.S. and Mackenzie D. 1982. "Immunospecific Ferromagnetic Iron Dextran Reagents for The Labelling and Magnetic Separation of Cells". *J. Immunol. Methods*, 52, 353–367.

51. Moore S. and Prevelige P. 2002. "DNA Packaging: A New Class of Molecular Motors". *Curr. Biol.*, 12, R96–R98.

52. Muldoon L.L., Tratnyek P.G., Jacobs P.M., Doolittle N.D., Christoforidis G.A., Frank J.A., Lindau M., Lockman P.R., Manninger S.P., Qiang Y., Spence A.M., Stupp S.I., Zhang M., and Neuwelt E.A. 2006. " Imaging and nanomedicine for diagnosis and therapy in the central nervous system: Report of the eleventh annual bloodbrain barrier disruption consortium meeting". *Am J Neuroradiol* 27: 715–721.

53. Muller R.H. and Keck C.M. 2004. "Challenges and Solutions for The Delivery of Biotech Drugs-A Review of Drug Nanocrystal Technology and Lipid Nanoparticles". *J. Biotechnol.*, 113, 151–170.

54. Na K. and Bae Y.H. 2002. "Self-Assembled Hydrogel Nanoparticles Responsive to Tumour Extracellular Ph From Pullulan Derivative/Sulphonamide Conjugate: Characterization, Aggregation and Adriamycin Release *In Vitro*". *Pharm. Res.*, 19, 681–683.

55. Nam J.M., Thaxton C.C. and Mirkin C.A. 2000. "Nanoparticles Based Bao-Bar Codes for The Ultrasensitive Detection of Proteins". *Science*, 301, 1884–1886.

56. Nishizawa M., Menon V.P. and Martin C.R. 1995. "Metal Nanotubule Membranes with Electrochemically Switchable Ion-Transport Selectivity". *Science*, 268, 700–702.

57. Panatarotto D., Prtidos C.D., Hoebeke J., Brown F., Kramer E., Briand J.P., Muller S., Prato M., and Bianco A. 2003. "Immunization with Peptide-Functionalized Carbon

Nanotubes Enhances Virus-Specific Neutralizing Antibody Responses". *Chemistry and Biology*, 10, 961–966.

58. Pohorille A. and Deamer D. 2002. "Artificial Cells: Prospects for Biotechnology". *Trends Biotechnol.*, 20, 123–128.

59. Quantum Dot Corporation web site accessed on April 20th 2005.

60. Reynolds A.R., Moein Moghimi S. and Hodivala-Dilke K. 2003. "Nanoparticle Mediated Gene Delivery to Tumour Neovasculature". *Trends Mol. Med.*, 9, 2–4.

61. Richard Feynman. 1963. "Six Easy Pieces", Addison-Wesley Pub. Co., Menlo Park, CA.

62. Rivas G. A., Miscoria S.A., Desbrieres J., and Barrera G.D. 2006. "New biosensing platforms based on the layer-by-layer self-assembling polyelectrolytes on Nafion/carbon nanotubes-coated glassy carbon electrodes". *Talanta* (in press, 2006).

63. Robert A. Freitas Jr. 1999. "Nanomedicine", Volume I: Basic Capabilities, Landes Bioscience, Georgetown, TX.

64. Roco M.C. 2001 "International Strategy for Nanotechnology Research and Development". *J. Nanoparticle Res.*, 3, 353–360.

65. Roy I., Mitra S., Maitra A. and Mozumdar S. 2003. "Calcium Phosphate Nanoparticles as Novel Non-Viral Vectors for Targeted Gene Delivery". *International Journal of Pharmaceutics*, 250, 25–33.

66. Roy I., Ohulchanskyy T.Y., Bharali D.J., Pudavar H.E., Mistretta R.A., Kaur N. and Prasad P.N. 2005. "Optical Tracking of Organically Modified Silica Nanoparticles as DNA Carriers: A Non-viral, Nanomedicine Approach for Gene Delivery". *PNAS*, 102 (2), 279–284.

67. Roy I., Ohulchanskyy T.Y., Pudavar H.E., et al. 2003. "Ceramic-Based Nanoparticles Entrapping Water-Insoluble Photosensitizing Anticancer Drugs: A Novel Drug-Carrier System for Photodynamic Therapy" *J. Am. Chem. Soc.*, 125, 7860–7865.

68. Sadeghi S.J., Tsotsou G.E., Fairhead M., Meharenna Y.T. and Gilardi G. 2001. "Rational Design of P450 Enzymes for Biotechnology" In: De Cuyper M., Bulte J. (Eds.), *Focus on Biotechnology.Physics and Chemistry Basis of Biotechnology*", Kluwer Academic Publisher, Dordrecht, 71–104.

69. Salem A.K., Hung C.F., Kim T.W., Wu T.C., Searson P.C. and Leong K.W. 2005. "Multi-Component Nanorods for Vaccination Applications". *Nanotechnology*, 16, 484–487.

70. Savage N and Diallo M. S. 2006. "Nanomaterials and water purification: opportunities and challenges". *J Nanoparticle Res* 7: 331–342.

71. Schaefer M. 2005. Double tightness. Lebensmitteltechnik 37: 52, 55.

72. Schwaneberg U., Schmidt Dannert C., Schmitt J. and Schmid R.D. 1999. "A Continuous Spectrophotometric Assay for P450 Bm3, A Fatty Acid Hydroxylating Enzyme and Its Mutant F87A". *Anal. Biochem.*, 269, 359–366.

73. Taniguchi N. 1974. "*On the Basic Concept of 'Nano-technology*". *Proc. Intl. Conf. Prod.* London, Part II British Society of Precision Engineering.

74. Thrall J. H. 2004 "*Nanotechnology and Medicine. Radiology*", Vol. 230(2), 315–318.

75. Tiefenauer L. and Ros R. 2002. "Biointerface Analysis on A Molecular Level: New Tools for Biosensor Research", Colloids Surfaces B. *Biointerfaces*, 23, 95–114.

76. Tsotsou G.E., Cass A.E.G and Gilardi G. 2002. "High Throughput Assay for P450 BM3 For Screening Libraries of Substrates and Combinatorial Mutants". *Biosens. Bioelectron.*, 17, 119–130.

77. Vohra A., Goswami D.Y., Deshpande D.A., and Block S.S. 2005. "Enhanced photocatalytic inactivation of bacterial spores on surfaces in air". *J Indust Microbiol Biotechnol* 32: 364–370.

78. Vohra A., Goswami D.Y., Deshpande D.A., and Block S.S. 2006. "Enhanced photocatalytic disinfection of indoor air". *Appl Catalysis B-Environ* 64:57–65.

79. Wang X., Li Y., Wei J. and de Groot K. 2002. "Development of Biomimetic Nano-hydroxyapatite/Poly (Hexamethylene Adipamide) Composites". *Biomaterials*, 23, 4787–4791.

80. Weissleder R., Elizondo G., Wittenburg J., Rabito C. A., Bengele H. H. and Josephson L. 1990. "Ultrasmall Superparamagnetic Iron Oxide:Characterization of a New Class of Contrast Agents for MR Imaging". *Radiology*, 175, 489–493.

81. Wen H.W., Borejsza-Wysocki W., DeCory T.R., Baeumner A.J., and Durst R.A. 2005. "A novel extraction method for peanut allergenic proteins in chocolate and their detection by a liposome-based lateral flow assay". *Eur Food Res Technol* 221: 564–569.

82. Wickline S.A., Neubauer A.M., Winter P., Caruthers S., and Lanza G. 2006. "Applications of nanotechnology to atherosclerosis, thrombosis, and vascular biology". *Arterioscler Thromb Vasc Biol* 26: 435–441.

83. Xu H., Aylott J.W., Kopelman R., Miller T.J. and Philbert M.A.2001. "A Real-Time Ratiometric Method for The Determination of Molecular Oxygen inside Living Cells Using Sol-Gel-Based Spherical Optical Nanosensors with Applications to Rat C6 Glioma". *Anal. Chem.*, 73, 4124–4133.

84. Yoshida J. and Kobayashi T. 1999. "Intracellular Hyperthermia for Cancer Using Magnetite Cationic Liposomes". *J. Magn. Mater.*, 194, 176–184.

85. Zhang Z.P and Feng S.S. 2006. "The drug encapsulation efficiency, in vitro drug release, cellular uptake and cytotoxicity of paclitaxel-loaded poly(lactide)- tocopheryl polyethylene glycol succinate nanoparticles". *Biomaterials* 27:4025–4033.

11

Application of Bioinformatics in Plant Science

Ashutosh Bahuguna • Madhuri K Lily • Koushalya Dangwal

INTRODUCTION

Recent developments in technologies and instrumentation, which allow large-scale as well as nano-scale probing of biological samples, are generating an exceptional amount of digital data. This sea of data is too much for the human brain to process and thus there is an increasing need to use computational methods to process and contextualize these data. Bioinformatics refers to the study of biological information using concepts and methods in computer science, statistics, and engineering. It can be divided into two categories — biological information management and computational biology. The National Institute of Health (NIH) (http://www.bisti.nih.gov/) defines the earlier category as "research, development, or application of computational tools and approaches for expanding the use of biological, medical, behavioral or health data, including those to acquire, represent, describe, store, analyze, or visualize such data." The second category is defined as "the development and application of data-analytical and theoretical methods, mathematical modeling, and computational simulation techniques to the study of biological, behavioral, and social systems." The boundaries of these categories are becoming more diffuse and other categories will no doubt surface in the future as this field matures.

This chapter introduces sequence-based analyses, including gene finding, gene family and phylogenetic analyses, and comparative genomics approaches, presents computational transcriptome analysis, ranging from analyses of various array technologies to regulatory sequence prediction, computational proteomics, including gel analysis and protein identification by mass-spectrometry data, computational metabolomics biological ontologies and their applications and various issues related to biological databases.

Sequence Analysis

Biological sequence such as DNA, RNA, and protein sequence is the most fundamental object for a biological system at the molecular level. Several genomes have been sequenced to a high quality in plants, including *Arabidopsis thaliana* (The Arabidopsis genome initiative, 2000 and rice Goff *et al.* 2002, Gibbs and Weinstock 2003, Yuj *et at.* 2002, Yuan *et al.* 2005). Draft genome sequences are available for poplar (http://genome. jgi-psf.org/Poptr1/) and lotus (http://www.kazusa.or.jp/lotus/), and sequencing efforts are in progress for several others including tomato, maize, *Medicago truncatula*, sorghum (Bedell *et al.* 2005) and close relatives of *Arabidopsis thaliana*. Researchers also generated expressed sequence tags (ESTs) from many plants including lotus, beet, soybean, cotton, wheat, and sorghum (*see* http://www.ncbi.nlm.nih.gov/dbEST/).

Genome Sequencing

Advances in sequencing technologies provide opportunities in bioinformatics for managing, processing, and analyzing the sequences. Shotgun sequencing is currently the most common method in genome sequencing: Pieces of DNA are sheared randomly, cloned and sequenced in parallel. Software has been developed to piece together the random, overlapping segments that are sequenced separately into a coherent and accurate contiguous sequence (Myers 1995). Numerous software packages exist for sequence assembly (Gibbs and Weinstock 2003), including Phred/ Phrap/Consed (http://www.phrap.org), Arachne (http://www.broad.mit.edu/wga/), and GAP4 (http://staden.sourceforge.net/overview.html). Current limitations in shotgun sequencing and assembly software remain largely in the assembly of highly repetitive sequences, although the cost of sequencing is another limitation. Recently developed methods continue to reduce the cost of sequencing, including sequencing by using differential hybridization of oligonucleotide probes (Frazer *et al.* 2003, Hinds *et al.* 2005, Patil *et al.* 2001), polymorphism ratio sequencing (Blazej *et al.* 2004), four-color DNA sequencing by synthesis on a chip (Seo *et al.* 2005). Each of these sequencing technologies has significant analytical challenges for bioinformatics in terms of experimental design, data interpretation, and analysis of the data in conjunction with other data.

Gene Finding and Genome Annotation

Gene finding refers to prediction of introns and exons in a segment of DNA sequence. Many of computer programs for identifying protein-coding genes are available. Some of the well-known ones include Genscan (http://genes.mit.edu/GENSCAN.html), GeneMarkHMM (http://opal.biology.gatech.edu/GeneMark/), GRAIL (http:// compbio.ornl.gov/Grail-1.3/), Genie (http://www.fruitfly.org/seqtools/genie.html), and Glimmer (http://www.tigr.org/softlab/glimmer). Several new gene-finding tools are modified for applications to plant genomic sequences (Schlueter *et al.* 2003). *Ab initio* (gene finding, in which genomic DNA sequence alone is systematically searched for certain tell-tale signs of protein-coding genes). These signs can be broadly categorized as either *signals*, specific sequences that indicate the presence of a gene nearby, or *content*, statistical properties of protein-coding sequence itself. *Ab initio* gene finding might be more accurately characterized as gene *prediction*, since extrinsic evidence is generally required to conclusively establish that a putative gene is functional, gene prediction remains a challenging problem, especially for large-sized eukaryotic genomes.

Sequence Comparison

Comparing sequences provides a foundation for many bioinformatic tools and may allow inference of the function, structure, and evolution of genes and genomes. For example, sequence comparison provides a basis for building a consensus gene model like UniGene (Blueggel *et al.* 2004). Also, many computational methods have been developed for homology identification (Wanx 2005). Although sequence comparison is highly useful, it should be noted that it is based on sequence similarity between two strings of text, which may not correspond to homology (relatedness to a common ancestor in evolution). Also, homology may not mean conservation in function. Methods in sequence comparison can be largely grouped into pair-wise, sequence profile, and profile-profile comparison. For pair-wise sequence comparison, FASTA (http://fasta.bioch.virginia.edu/) and BLAST (http://www.ncbi.nlm.nih.gov/blast/) are popular. Sequence-profile alignment is more sensitive for detecting remote homologs. A protein sequence profile is generated by multiple sequence alignment of a group of closely related proteins. A multiple sequence alignment builds correspondence among residues across all of the sequences simultaneously, where aligned positions in different sequences probably show functional and/or structural relationship. A sequence profile is calculated using the probability of occurrence for each amino acid at each alignment position. PSI-BLAST (http://www.ncbi.nlm.nih.gov/BLAST/) is a popular example of a sequence-profile alignment tool. Some other sequence-profile comparison methods are slower but even more accurate than PSI-BLAST, including HMMER (http://hmmer.wustl.edu/), SAM (http://www.cse.ucsc.edu/research/compbio/sam.html), and META-MEME (http://metameme.sdsc.edu/). A profile-profile alignment is more sensitive than the sequence profile-based search programs in detecting remote homologs. However, due to its high false positive rate, profile-profile comparison is not widely used. Given potential false positive predictions, it is helpful to correlate the sequence comparison results with the relationship observed in functional genomic data.

TRANSCRIPTOME ANALYSIS

The primary goal of transcriptome analysis is to learn about how changes in transcript abundance control growth and development of an organism and its response to the environment. DNA microarrays proved a powerful technology for observing the transcriptional profile of genes at a genome-wide level (Brown and Botstein 1999, Schena *et al.* 1995). Microarray data are also being combined with other information such as regulatory sequence analysis, gene ontology, and pathway information to infer coregulated processes. Whole-genome tiled arrays are used to detect transcription without bias toward known or predicted gene structures and alternative splice variants.

Microarray Analysis

Microarray analysis allows the simultaneous measurement of transcript abundance for thousands of genes (Zhu, Wang 2000). Two general types of microarrays are high-density oligonucleotide arrays that contain a large number (thousands or often millions) of relatively short (25–100-mer) probes synthesized directly on the surface of the arrays, or arrays with amplified polymerase chain reaction products or cloned DNA fragments mechanically spotted directly on the array surface. Many different technologies are being developed, which have been recently surveyed by Meyers and colleagues. Competition among microarray platforms has led to lower costs and increased numbers of genes per array. Unfortunately, the diversity of array platforms makes it difficult to compare results between microarray formats that use different probe sequences, RNA sample labeling, and data collection methods (Woo *et al.* 2004). Other important issues in microarray analysis are in processing and normalizing data. Some journals require multiple biological replicates (typically at least three) and statistically valid results before publishing microarray results. Replication of the microarray experiment and appropriate statistical design are needed to minimize the false discovery rate. The microarray data must also be deposited into a permanent public repository with open access. The main difficulty of dealing with microarray data is the sheer amount of data resulting from a single experiment. This makes it very difficult to decide which transcripts to focus on for interpreting the results.

Even for standardized arrays such as those from Affymetrix, there are still arguments on the optimal statistical treatment for the sets of probes designed for each gene. For example, the *Affycomp* software compares Affymetrix results using two spike-in experiments and a dilution experiment for different methods of normalization under different assessment criteria (Cope *et al.* 2004). This information can be used to select the appropriate normalization methods. Many tools are available that perform a variety of analysis on large microarray data sets. Examples include commercial software such as Gene Traffic, GeneSpring (http://www.agilent.com/chem/genespring), Affymetrix's GeneChip Operating Software (GCOS), and public software such as Cluster (Eisen *et al.* 1998, CaARRAY (http://caarray.nci.nih.gov/), and BASE (Brown and Sansean 2005, Boguski *et al.* 1995, Goff *et al.* 2002).

Tiling Arrays

Typical microarray sample known and predicted genes. Tiling arrays cover the genome at regular intervals to measure transcription without bias toward known or predicted gene structures, discovery of polymorphisms, analysis of alternative splicing, and identification of transcription factor-binding sites (Muckler and Ecker 2005). Whole-genome arrays (WGAs) cover the entire genome with overlapping probes or probes with regular gaps. The WGA ensures that the experimental results are not dependent on the level of current genome annotation as well as discovering new transcripts and unusual forms of transcription. In plants, similar studies have been performed for the entire *Arabidopsis* genome (Stok *et al.* 2005, Yamada 2003) and parts of the rice genome (Li *et al.* 1998). These studies identified thousands of novel transcription units including genes within the centromeres, substantial antisense gene transcription, and transcription activity in intergenic regions. Tiling array data may also be used to validate predicted intron/exon boundaries (Toyoda and Shizozaki 2005).

Regulatory Sequence Analysis

Interpreting the results of microarray experiments involves discovering why genes with similar expression profiles behave in a coordinated fashion. Regulatory sequence analysis approaches this question by extracting motifs that are shared between the upstream sequences of these genes (Van Helden, 2003). Comparative genomics studies of conserved noncoding sequences (CNSs) may also help to find key motifs (Inada *et al.* 2003). There are several methods to search over-represented motifs at the upstream of coregulated genes. Roughly, they can be categorized into two classes—oligonucleotide frequency-based (Jensen and Knudsen 2000, Van Helden 2003) and probabilistic sequence-based models (Lawrence 1993, Marchal 2003, Roth *et al.* 1998). The oligonucleotide frequency-based method calculates the statistical significance of a site based on oligonucleotide frequency tables observed in all noncoding regions of the specific organism's genome. Usually, the length of the oligonucleotide varies from 4 to 9 bases. Hexanucleotide (oligonucleotide length of 6) analysis is most widely used. The significant oligonucleotides can then be grouped as longer consensus motifs. Frequency-based methods tend to be simple, efficient, and exhaustive (all over-represented patterns of chosen length are detected). The main limitation is the difficulty of identifying complex motif patterns. The public Web resource, Regulatory Sequence Analysis Tools (RSAT), performs sequence similarity searches and analyzes the noncoding sequences in the genomes (Van Helden, 2003). For the probabilistic-based methods, the motif is represented as a position probability matrix, where the motifs are assumed to be hidden in the noisy background sequences.

One of the strengths of probabilistic-based methods is the ability to identify motifs with complex patterns. Many potential motifs can be identified; however, it can be difficult to separate unique motifs from this large pool of potential solutions. Probabilistic-based methods also tend to be computationally intense as they must be run multiple times to get an optimal solution. AlignACE, Aligns Nucleic Acid Conserved Elements (http://atlas.med.harvard.edu/), is a popular motif finding tool that was first developed for yeast but has been expanded to other species (Roberts *et al.* 2000).

COMPUTATIONAL PROTEOMICS

Proteomics is a leading technology for the qualitative and quantitative characterization of proteins and their interactions on a genome scale. The objectives of proteomics include large-scale identification and quantification of all protein types in a cell or tissue, analysis of post-translational modification and association with other proteins, and characterization of protein activities and structures. Application of proteomics in plants is still in its initial phase, mostly in protein identification. Other aspects of proteomics (Zhu *et al.* 2003), such as identification and prediction of protein-protein interactions, protein activity profiling, protein subcellular localization, and protein structure, have not been widely used in plant science. However, recent efforts such as the structural genomic initiative that includes *Arabidopsis* (http://www.uwstructuralgenomics.org/) are encouraging.

Electrophoresis Analysis

Electrophoresis analysis can qualitatively and quantitatively investigate expression of proteins under different conditions (Gorg *et al.* 2000). Several bioinformatics tools have been developed for two-dimensional (2D) electrophoresis analysis (Marengo *et al.* 2003). SWISS-2DPAGE can locate the proteins on the 2D PAGE maps from Swiss-Prot (http://au.expasy.org/ch2d/). Melanie (http://au.expasy.org/melanie/) can analyze, annotate, and query complex 2D gel samples. Flicker (http://open2dprot.sourceforge.net/Flicker/) is an open-source stand-alone program for visually comparing 2D gel images. PDQuest (http://www.proteomeworks.bio-rad.com) is a popular commercial software package for comparing 2D gel images.

Protein Identification through Mass Spectrometry

After protein separation using 2D electrophoresis or liquid chromatography and protein digestion using an enzyme (trypsin, pepsin, glu-C, etc.), proteins are identified by typically using mass spectrometry (MS; Ashburner, 2000). In contrast to other protein identification techniques, such as Edman degradation microsequencing, MS provides a high-throughput approach for large-scale protein identification. The data generated from mass spectrometers are often complicated and computational analyses are critical in interpreting the data for protein identification (Blueggel *et al.* 2004, Grass Muller 2001). A major limitation in MS protein identification is the lack of open-source software. Most widely used tools are expensive commercial packages. In addition, current statistical models for matches between MS spectra and protein sequences are generally oversimplified. Hence, the confidence assessments for computational protein identification results are often unreliable. There are two types of MS-based protein identification methods—peptide mass fingerprinting (PMF) and tandem mass spectrometry (MS/MS).

Peptide Mass Fingerprinting

PMF peptide/protein identification compares the masses of peptides derived from the experimental spectral peaks with each of the possible peptides computationally digested from proteins in the sequence database. The proteins in the sequence database with a significant number of peptide matches are considered candidates for the proteins in the experimental sample. MOWSE was an earlier software package for PMF protein identification, and Emowse (http://emboss.sourceforge.net/) is the latest implementation of the MOWSE algorithm. Several other computational tools have also been developed for PMF protein identification. MS-Fit in the Protein Prospector (http://prospector.ucsf.edu/) uses a variant of MOWSE scoring scheme incorporating new features, including constraints on the minimum number of peptides to be matched for a possible hit.

Tandem Mass Spectrometry

MS/MS further breaks each digested peptide into smaller fragments, whose spectra provide effective signatures of individual amino acids in the peptide for protein identification. Many tools have been developed for MS/MS-based peptide/protein identification, the most popular ones being SEQUEST http://fields.scripps.edu/sequest/) and Mascot (http://www.matrixscience.com/). Both rely on the comparison between theoretical peptides derived from the database and experimental mass spectrometric tandem spectra.

METABOLOMICS AND METABOLIC FLUX

Metabolomics is the analysis of the complete pool of small metabolites in a cell at any given time. Metabolomics may prove to be particularly important in plants due to the proliferation of secondary metabolites. As of 2004, more than 100,000 metabolites have been identified in plants, with estimates that this may be less than 10% of the total (Trethewey, 2004). In a metabolite profiling experiment, metabolites are extracted from tissues, separated, and analyzed in a high-throughput manner (Fiehn 2002). Metabolic fingerprinting looks at a few metabolites to help differentiate samples according to their phenotype or biological relevance (Harrigan and Goodacre 2003, Shanks 2005). Technology has now advanced to semi-automatically quantify >1000 compounds from a single leaf extract. The key challenge in metabolite profiling is the rapid, consistent, and unambiguous identification of metabolites from complex plant samples. Identification is routinely performed by time-consuming standard addition experiments using commercially available or purified metabolite preparations. A publicly accessible database that contains the evidence and underlying metabolite identification for gas chromatography-mass spectrometry (GC–MS) profiles from diverse biological sources is needed. Standards for experimental metadata and data quality in metabolomics experiments are still in a very early stage and a large-scale public repository is not yet available. The ArMet (architecture for metabolomics) proposal gives a description of plant metabolomics experiments and their results along with a database schema. MIAMET (minimum information about a metabolomics experiment) (Bino *et al.* 2004) gives reporting requirements with the aim of standardizing experiment descriptions, particularly within publications. The standard metabolic reporting structures (SMRS) working group (SMRS working group; 2005) has developed standards for describing the biological sample origin, analytical technologies, and methods used in a metabolite profiling experiment. Metabolite data have been used to construct metabolic correlation networks (Steuer *et al.* 2003). Such correlations may reflect the net partitioning of carbon and nitrogen resulting from direct enzymatic conversions and indirect cellular regulation by transcriptional or biochemical processes. However, metabolic correlation matrices cannot infer that a change in one metabolite led to a change in another metabolite in a metabolic reaction network (Steuer *et al.* 2003). Metabolic flux analysis measures the steady-state flow between metabolites. Fluxes, however, are even more difficult to measure than metabolite levels due to complications in modeling intracellular transport of metabolites and the incomplete knowledge about the topology and location of the pathways in vivo (Shanks, 2005). The most basic approach to metabolic flux analysis is stoichiometric analysis that calculates the quantities of reactants and products of a chemical reaction to determine the flux of each metabolite. However, this method is numerically difficult to solve for large networks and it has problems, if parallel metabolic pathways, metabolic cycles, and reversible reactions are present (Wiechart *et al.* 2001). Flux-Analyzer is a package for MATLAB that integrates pathway and flux analysis for metabolic networks (Klamt *et al.* 2003). Flux analysis using ^{13}C carbon labelling data seeks to overcome some of the disadvantages of stoichiometric flux analysis described above (Sriram *et al.* 2004). More rigorous analysis is needed for full determination of fluxes from all of the experimental data in ^{13}C constrained flux analysis (stoichiometric model with a few flux ratios as constraints) and the stoichiometric and isotopomer balances. Iterative methods have been used to solve the resulting matrix of isotopomer balances, with the nuclear magnetic resonance or gas chromatography measurements used to provide consistency. As more reliable data are collected, one can use ordinary differential equations for dynamic simulations of metabolic networks and combine information about connectivity, concentration balances, flux balances, metabolic control, and pathway optimization. Ultimately, one may integrate all of the information and perform analysis and simulation in a cellular modeling environment like E-Cell (http://www.e-cell.org/) or Cell Designer (http://www.systems-biology.org).

ONTOLOGIES

The data that are generated and analyzed as described in the previous sections need to be compared with the existing knowledge in the field in order to place the data in a biologically meaningful context and derive hypotheses. To do this efficiently, data and knowledge need to be described in explicit and unambiguous ways that must be comprehensible to both humans and computer programs. Ontology is a set of vocabulary terms whose meanings and relations with other terms are explicitly stated and which are used to annotate data (Ashburner *et al.* 2000, Bard *et al.* 2005, Blake 2004, Stevens 2000). This section introduces the types of ontologies in development and use today and some applications and caveats of using the ontologies in biology.

Types of Bio-ontologies

A growing number of shared ontologies are being built and used in biology. Examples include ontologies for describing gene and protein function (Harris *et al.* 2004), cell types (Bard *et al.* 2005), anatomies and developmental stages of organisms (Garcia *et al.* 2002) microarray experiments (Ware *et al.* 2002) and metabolic pathways (Maox *et al.* 2005). A list of open-source ontologies used in biology can be found on the Open Biological Ontologies Web site (http://obo.sourceforge.net/). Much ontologies on this site are under development and are subject to frequent change. The Gene Ontology (GO) (www.geneontology.org) is an example of bio-ontologies that has garnered community acceptance. It is a set of more than 16,000 controlled vocabulary terms for the biological domains of "molecular function," "subcellular compartment," and "biological process".

DATABASES

Traditionally, biologists relied on textbooks and research articles published in scientific journals as the main source of information. This has changed dramatically in the past decade as the Internet and Web browsers became commonplace. Today, the Internet is the first place researchers go to find information. Databases that are available via the Web also became an indispensable tool for biological research. In this section, we describe types and examples of biological databases, how these databases are built and accessed, how data among databases are exchanged, and current challenges and opportunities in biological database development and maintenance.

Types of Biological Databases

Three types of biological databases have been established and are developed — large scale public repositories, community-specific databases, and project-specific databases.

Nucleic Acids Research (http://nar.oxfordjournals.org/) publishes a database issue in January of every year. Recently, *Plant Physiology* started publishing articles describing databases (Rhee Crosby, 2005). Large-scale public repositories are usually developed and maintained by government agencies or international consortia and are places for long-term data storage. Examples include GenBank for sequences, UniProt (Rhee *et al.* 2005) for protein information, Protein Data Bank for protein structure information, and Array Express and Gene Expression Omnibus (GEO) (Edgar *et al.* 2002) for microarray data. There are a number of community-specific databases, which typically contain information curated with high standards and address the needs of a particular community of researchers. A prominent example of community-specific databases is those that cater to researchers focused on studying model organisms or clade-oriented comparative databases (Gonzales *et al.* 2005, Mattenes *et al.* 2003, Muller *et al.* 2005, Ware *et al.* 2002). Other examples of community-specific databases include databases focused on specific types of data such as metabolism and protein modification (Tchieu *et al.* 2003). The concept of community-specific databases is subject to change as researchers are widening their scope of research. For example, databases focused on comparing genome sequences recently emerged (e.g. http://www.phytome.org and Horan *et al.* 2006). The third category of databases includes smaller-scale, and often short-lived, databases that are developed for project data management during the funding period.

Data Representation and Storage

Databases can be developed using a number of different methods including simple file directories, object-oriented database software, and relational database software. Due to the increasing quantity of data that need to be stored and made accessible using the Internet, relational database management software has become popular and has become the de facto standard in biology. Relational databases provide effective means of storing and retrieving large quantities of data via indexes, normalization, referential integrity, triggers, and transactions. Notable relational database software that is freely available and quite popular in bioinformatics is My SQL (http://www.mysql.com/) and Postgre SQL (http://www.postgresql.org/).

Data Access and Exchange

The most direct, powerful, and flexible way of accessing data in a database is using structured query language (SQL) (http://databases.about.com/od/sql/). SQL has a reasonably intuitive and simple syntax that requires no programming knowledge and issuited for biologists to learn without a steep learning curve. However, to use SQL, users need to know the database schema. In addition, some queries that are based on less optimized database structure could result in slow performance and can even sometimes lock the database system. In most databases, access to the data is provided via database access software and graphical user interface (GUI) that allow searching and browsing of the data. In addition to text-based search user interfaces, more sophisticated ways of accessing data such as graphical displays and tree-based browsers are also common.

Data Curation

Data curation is defined as any activity devoted to selecting, organizing, assessing quality, describing, and updating data that result in enhanced quality, trustworthiness, interpretability, and longevity of the data. It is a crucial task in today's research environment where data are being generated at an ever increasing rate and an increasing amount of research is based on re-use of data. In general, some level of curation is done by data generators, but most curation activities are carried out in data repositories. A number of different strategies to curation are used, including computational, manual, in-house, and those that involve external expertise. Assessing data quality involves both determining the criteria for measuring quality and performing the measurements. Data quality criteria for raw data are tied with methods of data acquisition. In many databases, these criteria are not made explicit and the information on the metrics of data-quality assessment is rare. Curation of data into public repositories should be a parallel and integrated process with publication in peer-reviewed journals. Although much progress has been made in electronic publication and open-access publishing, there is still a gap between connecting the major conclusions in papers and the data that were used to draw the conclusions. In a few cases, data are required to be submitted to public repositories (e.g. sequence data to GenBank, microarray data to Array-Express/GEO, and *Arabidopsis* stock data to ABRC). However, there are no such standards established for other data types (e.g. proteomics data, metabolomics data, protein localization, in situ hybridization, phenotype description, protein function information). Standards, specifications, and requirements for publication of data into repositories should be made more accessible to researchers early on in their data-generation and research activity processes. One of the most important aspects of today's changing research landscape is the culture of data and expertise sharing. The now famous Bermuda principle (http://www.gene.ucl.ac.uk/hugo/bermuda.htm).

EMERGING AREAS IN BIOINFORMATICS

In addition to some of the challenges and opportunities mentioned in this article, there are many exciting areas of research in bioinformatics that are emerging, few of these areas such as text mining, systems biology, and the semantic web. Some additional emerging areas such as image analysis, grid computing, directed evolution, rational protein design, microRNA-related bioinformatics, and modeling in epigenomics.

REFERENCE

1. Ashburner M, Ball C, Blake J *et al*. 2000. Gene ontology: tool for the unification of biology. *The Gene Ontology Consortium. Nat. Genet*. 25:25–29.

2. Bard J, Rhee SY, Ashburner M. 2005. An ontology for cell types. *Genome Biol*. 6:R21.

3. Bard JB, Rhee SY. 2004. Ontologies in biology: design, applications and future challenges. *Nat. Rev. Genet*. 5:213–22.

4. Bedell JA, Budiman MA, Nunberg A, et al. 2005. Sorghum genome sequencing by methylation filtration. *PLoS Biol*. 3:e13.

5. Bino R, Hall R, Fiehn O, Kopka J and Saito K, 2004. Potential of metabolomics as a functional genomics tool. *Trends Plant Sci*. 9:418–25.

6. Blake J. 2004. Bio-ontologies-fast and furious. *Nat. Biotechnol.* 22:773–74.

7. Blazej RG, Paegel BM and Mathies RA. 2003. Polymorphism ratio sequencing: a new approach for single nucleotide polymorphism discovery and genotyping. *Genome Res.* 13:287–93.

8. Blueggel M, Chamrad D and Meyer HE. 2004. Bioinformatics in proteomics. *Curr. Pharm. Biotechnol.* 5:79–88.

9. Boguski MS and Schuler GD. 1995. ESTablishing a human transcript map. *Nat. Genet.* 10:369–71.

10. Brown JR and Sanseau P. 2005. A computational view of microRNAs and their targets. *Drug Discov. Today* 10:595–601.

11. Brown P and Botstein D. 1999. Exploring the new world of the genome with DNA microarrays. *Nat. Genet.* 21:33–37.

12. Cope LM, Irizarry RA, Jaffee HA, Wu Z and Speed TP. 2004. A benchmark for Affymetrix GeneChip expression measures. *Bioinformatics* 20:323–31.

13. Edgar R, Domrachev M and Lash AE. 2002. Gene Expression Omnibus: NCBI gene expression and hybridization array data repository. *Nucleic Acids. Res.* 30:207–10 a tool for the unification of genome annotations. *Genome Biol.* 6:R44.

14. Eisen MB, Spellman PT, Brown PO and Botstein D. 1998. Cluster analysis and display of genome-wide expression patterns. *Proc. Natl. Acad. Sci.* USA 95:14863–68.

15. Fiehn O. 2002. Metabolomics—the link between genotypes and phenotypes. *Plant Mol. Biol.* 48:155–71.

16. Frazer KA, Chen X, Hinds DA, Pant PV, Patil N and Cox DR. 2003. Genomic DNA insertions and deletions occur frequently between humans and nonhuman primates. *Genome Res.* 13:341–46.

17. Garcia-Hernandez M, Berardini TZ, Chen G, Crist D and Doyle A, *et al*. 2002. TAIR: a resource for integrated Arabidopsis data. *Funct. Integr. Genomics* 2:239–53.

18. Gibbs RA and Weinstock GM. 2003. Evolving methods for the assembly of large genomes. Cold Spring Harb. *Symp. Quant. Biol.* 68:189–94.

19. Goff SA, Ricke D, Lan TH, Presting G and Wang R, *et al*. 2002. A draft sequence of the rice genome (Oryza sativa L. ssp. japonica). *Science* 296:92–100.

20. Gonzales MD, Archuleta E, Farmer A, Gajendran K and Grant D, 2005. The Legume Information System (LIS): an integrated information resource for comparative legume biology. *Nucleic Acids Res.* 33:D660–65.

21. Gorg A, Obermaier C, Boguth G, Harder A and Scheibe B, *et al*. 2000. The current state of two-dimensional electrophoresis with immobilized pH gradients. *Electrophoresis* 21:1037–53.

22. Gras R, and Muller M. 2001. Computational aspects of protein identification by mass spectrometry. *Curr. Opin. Mol. Ther.* 3:526–32.

23. Harrigan GG, and Goodacre R, eds. 2003. *Metabolic Profiling: Its Role in Biomarker Discovery and Gene Function Analysis.* Boston: Plenum.

24. Harris MA, Clark J, Ireland A, Lomax J, and Ashburner M, 2004. The Gene Ontology (GO) database and informatics resource. *Nucleic Acids Res.* 32:D258–61.

25. Hinds DA, Stuve LL, Nilsen GB, Halperin E, and Eskin E, 2005. Whole-genome patterns of common DNA variation in three human populations. *Science* 307:1072–79.

26. Horan K, Lauricha J, Bailey-Serres J, Raikhel N, and Girke T. 2005. Genome cluster database. A sequence family analysis platform for Arabidopsis and rice. *Plant Physiol.* 138:47–54.

27. Inada DC, Bashir A, Lee C, Thomas BC, and Ko C, 2003. Conserved noncoding sequences in the grasses. *Genome Res.* 13:2030–41.

28. Jensen LJ, and Knudsen S. 2000. Automatic discovery of regulatory patterns in promoter regions based on whole cell expression data and functional annotation. *Bioinformatics* 16:326–33.

29. Klamt S, Stelling J, Ginkel M, and Gilles ED. 2003. FluxAnalyzer: exploring structure, pathways, and flux distributions in metabolic networks on interactive flux maps. *Bioinformatics* 19:261–69.

30. Lawrence CE, Altschul SF, Boguski MS, Liu JS, Neuwald AF, and Wootton JC. 1993. Detecting subtle sequence signals: a Gibbs sampling strategy for multiple alignment. *Science* 262:208–14.

31. Lewin B. 2003. *Genes VIII*. Upper Saddle River, NJ: Prentice Hall.

32. Li L, Wang X, Xia M, Stolc V, and Su N, *et al.* 2005. Tiling microarray analysis of rice chromosome 10 to identify the transcriptome and relate its expression to chromosomal architecture. *Genome Biol.* 6:R52.

33. Mao X, Cai T, Olyarchuk JG, and Wei L. 2005. Automated genome annotation and pathway identification using the KEGG Orthology (KO) as a controlled vocabulary. *Bioinformatics* 21:3787–93.

34. Marchal K, Thijs G, De Keersmaecker S, Monsieurs P, De Moor B, and Vanderleyden J. 2003. Genome-specific higher-order background models to improve motif detection. *Trends Microbiol.* 11:61–66.

35. Marengo E, Robotti E, Antonucci F, Cecconi D, Campostrini N, and Righetti PG. 2005. Numerical approaches for quantitative analysis of two-dimensional maps: a review of commercial software and home-made systems. *Proteomics* 5:654–66.

36. Matthews DE, Carollo VL, Lazo GR, and Anderson OD. 2003. GrainGenes, the genome database for small-grain crops. *Nucleic Acids Res.* 31:183–86.

37. Mockler TC, and Ecker JR. 2005. Applications of DNA tiling arrays for whole-genome analysis. *Genomics* 85:1–15.

38. Mueller LA, Solow TH, Taylor N, Skwarecki B, and Buels R, 2005. The SOL Genomics Network. A comparative resource for solanaceae biology and beyond. *Plant Physiol.* 138:1310–17.

39. Myers EW. 1995. Toward simplifying and accurately formulating fragment assembly. *J. Comput. Biol.* 2:275–90.

40. Parkinson H, Sarkans U, Shojatalab M, Abeygunawardena N, and Contrino S, 2005. Array Express — a public repository for microarray gene expression data at the EBI. *Nucleic Acids Res.* 33:D553–55.

41. Patil N, Berno AJ, Hinds DA, Barrett WA, and Doshi JM, 2001. Blocks of limited haplotype diversity revealed by high-resolution scanning of human chromosome 21. *Science* 294:1719–23.

42. Rhee SY, and Crosby B. 2005. Biological databases for plant research. *Plant Physiol.* 138:1–3.

43. Roberts C, Nelson B, Marton M, Stoughton R, and Meyer M, 2000. Signaling and circuitry of multiple MAPK pathways revealed by a matrix of global gene expression profiles. *Science* 287:873–80.

44. Roth FP, Hughes JD, Estep PW, and Church GM. 1998. Finding DNA regulatory motifs within unaligned noncoding sequences clustered by whole-genome mRNA quantitation. *Nat. Biotechnol.* 16:939–45.

45. Schena M, Shalon D, Davis RW, and Brown PO. 1995. Quantitative monitoring of gene expression patterns with a complementary DNA microarray. *Science* 270:467–70.

46. Schlueter SD, Dong Q, and Brendel V. 2003. GeneSeqer@PlantGDB: gene structure prediction in plant genomes. *Nucleic Acids Res.* 31:3597–600.

47. Schneider M, Bairoch A, Wu CH, and Apweiler R. 2005. Plant protein annotation in the UniProt Knowledgebase. *Plant Physiol.* 138:59–66.

48. Seo TS, Bai X, Kim DH, Meng Q, Shi S, *et al.* 2005. Four-color DNA sequencing by synthesis on a chip using photocleavable fluorescent nucleotides. *Proc. Natl. Acad. Sci. USA* 102:5926–31.

49. Shanks JV. 2005. Phytochemical engineering: combining chemical reaction engineering with plant science. *AIChE J.* 51:2–7.

50. SMRS Working Group. 2005. Summary recommendations for standardization and reporting of metabolic analyses. *Nat. Biotechnol.* 23:833–38.

51. Sriram G, Fulton DB, Iyer VV, Peterson JM, and Zhou R, 2004. Quantification of compartmented metabolic fluxes in developing soybean embryos by employing biosynthetically directed fractional ^{13}C labeling, two-dimensional [^{13}C, ^{1}H] nuclear magnetic resonance, and comprehensive isotopomer balancing. *Plant Physiol.* 136:3043–57.

52. Steuer R, Kurths J, Fiehn O, and Weckwerth W. 2003. Interpreting correlations in metabolomic networks. *Biochem. Soc. Trans.* 31:1476–78.

53. Steuer R, Kurths J, Fiehn O, and Weckwerth W. 2003. Observing and interpreting correlations in metabolomic networks. *Bioinformatics* 19:1019–26.

54. Stevens R, Goble CA, and Bechhofer S. 2000. Ontology-based knowledge representation for bioinformatics. *Brief Bioinform.* 1:398–414.

55. Stoeckert CJ Jr, Causton HC, and Ball CA. 2002. Microarray databases: standards and ontologies. *Nat. Genet.* 32 (Suppl.): 469–73.

56. Stolc V, Samanta MP, Tongprasit W, Sethi H, and Liang S, *et al.* 2005. Identification of transcribed sequences in Arabidopsis thaliana by using high-resolution genome tiling arrays. *Proc. Natl. Acad. Sci. USA* 102:4453–58.

57. Tchieu JH, Fana F, Fink JL, Harper J, and Nair TM, 2003. The PlantsP and PlantsT Functional Genomics Databases. *Nucleic Acids Res.* 31:342–44.

58. The Arabidopsis Genome Initiative. 2000. Analysis of the genome sequence of the flowering plant Arabidopsis thaliana. *Nature* 408:796–815.

59. Toyoda T, and Shinozaki K. 2005. Tiling array-driven elucidation of transcriptional structures based on maximum-likelihood and Markov models. *Plant J.* 43:611–21.

60. Trethewey R. 2004. Metabolite profiling as an aid to metabolic engineering in plants. *Curr. Opin. Plant Biol.* 7:196–201.

61. Van Helden J. 2003. Regulatory sequence analysis tools. Nucleic Acids Res. 31:3593–96.

62. Vincent PL, Coe EH, and Polacco ML. 2003. Zea mays ontology — a database of international terms. *Trends Plant Sci.* 8:517–20.

63. Wan X, and Xu D. 2005. Computational methods for remote homolog identification. *Curr. Protein Peptide Sci.* 6:527–46.

64. Ware DH, Jaiswal P, Ni J, Yap IV, and Pan X, *et al.* 2002. Gramene, a tool for grass genomics. *Plant Physiol.* 130:1606–13.

65. Wiechert W, Mollney M, Petersen S, and de Graaf AA. 2001. A universal framework for ^{13}C metabolic flux analysis. *Metab. Eng.* 3:265–83.

66. Woo Y, Affourtit J, Daigle S, Viale A, and Johnson K, 2004. A comparison of cDNA, oligonucleotide, and affymetrix GeneChip gene expression microarray platforms. *J. Biomol. Tech.* 15:276–84.

67. Yamada K, Lim J, Dale JM, Chen H, and Shinn P, 2003. Empirical analysis of transcriptional activity in the Arabidopsis genome. *Science* 302:842–46.

68. Yu J, Hu S, Wang J, Wong GK, and Li S, *et al.* 2002. A draft sequence of the rice genome (Oryza sativa L. ssp. indica). *Science* 296:79–92.

69. Yuan Q, Ouyang S, Wang A, Zhu W, and Maiti R, 2005. The institute for genomic research Osa1 rice genome annotation database. *Plant Physiol.* 138:18–26.

70. Zhang P, Foerster H, Tissier CP, Mueller L, and Paley S, 2005. MetaCyc and AraCyc. Metabolic pathway databases for plant research. *Plant Physiol.* 138:27–37.

71. Zhu H, Bilgin M, and Snyder M. 2003. Proteomics. *Annu. Rev. Biochem.* 72:783–812.

72. Zhu T, and Wang X. 2000. Large-scale profiling of the Arabidopsis transcriptome. *Plant Physiol.* 124:1472–76.

12

Gene Diversity and Emergence of Genome Evolution

Padma Singh • Bhavya Trivedi

INTRODUCTION

Gene is the fundamental, physical, and functional unit of heredity. It is because a gene is a segment of DNA (on a specific site on a chromosome) that is responsible for the physical and inheritable characteristics or phenotype of an organism. It also specifies the structure of a protein, and an RNA molecule. A gene is formerly called a factor. In modern molecular biology and genetics, the genome is the entirety of an organism's hereditary information. It is encoded either in DNA or, for many types of virus, in RNA. The genome includes both the genes and the non-coding sequences of the DNA/RNA. The term genome can be applied specifically to mean that stored on a complete set of nuclear DNA (i.e. the "nuclear genome") but can also be applied to that stored within organelles that contain their own DNA, as with the "mitochondrial genome" or the "chloroplast genome". Additionally, the genome can comprise nonchromosomal genetic elements such as viruses, plasmids, and transposable elements. The study of the global properties of genomes of related organisms is usually referred to as genomics, which distinguishes it from genetics which generally studies the properties of single genes or groups of genes. Complete genome sequences have served to define and to describe many genes and regulatory features as well as numerous other elements. They have also revealed the actions of gene gain, loss and rearrangement, and have shed light on the scope and impact of numerous genetic diversity and evolutionary processes.

Genetic diversity, the level of biodiversity, refers to the total number of genetic characteristics in the genetic makeup of a species. It is distinguished from genetic variability, which describes the tendency of genetic characteristics to vary.

Genetic diversity serves as a way for populations to adapt to changing environments. With more variation, it is more likely that some individuals in a population will possess variations of alleles that are suited for the environment. Those individuals are more likely to survive to produce offspring bearing that allele. The population will continue for more generations because of the success of these individuals. There are many different ways to measure genetic diversity. The modern causes for the loss of animal genetic diversity have also been studied and identified (Groom et al., 2006; Tisdell, 2003). A 2007 study conducted by the National Science Foundation found that genetic diversity and biodiversity are dependent upon each other—that diversity within a species is necessary to maintain diversity among species, and vice versa. According to the lead researcher in the study, Lankau, "If any one type is removed from the system, the cycle can breakdown, and the community becomes dominated by a single species."

Measures of Genetic Diversity

Genetic diversity of a population can be assessed by some simple measures:
- Gene diversity is the proportion of polymorphic loci across the genome.
- Heterozygosity is the mean number of individuals with polymorphic loci.
- Alleles per locus is also used to demonstrate variability.

Role of Genetic Diversity in Genome Evolution

Evolution requires genetic variation. If there were no dark moths, the population could not have evolved from mostly light to mostly dark. In order for continuing evolution, there must be mechanisms to increase or create genetic variation and mechanisms to decrease it. Mutation is a change in a gene. These changes are the source of new genetic variation. Natural selection operates on this variation.

Genetic variation has two components—allelic diversity and non-random associations of alleles. Alleles are different versions of the same gene. For example, humans can have A, B or O alleles that determine one aspect of their blood type. Most animals, including humans, are diploid—they contain two alleles for every gene at every locus, one inherited from their mother and one inherited from their father. Locus is the location of a gene on a chromosome. Humans can be AA, AB, AO, BB, BO or OO at the blood group locus. If the two alleles at a locus are the same type (for instance two A alleles), the individual would be called homozygous. An individual with two different alleles at a locus (e.g. an AB individual) is called heterozygous. At any locus, there can be many different alleles in a population, more alleles than any single organism can possess. For example, no single human can have an A, B and an O allela.

The non-random association is maintained by natural selection. Bright, tailed moths mimic the pattern of an unpalatable species. The dark morph is cryptic. The other two combinations are neither mimetic nor cryptic and are quickly eaten by birds. Assortative mating causes a non-random distribution of alleles at a single locus. (locus: location of a gene on a chromosome.) If there are two alleles (A and a) at a locus with frequencies p and q, the frequency of the three possible genotypes (AA, Aa and aa) will be p^2, $2pq$ and q^2, respectively. For example, if the frequency of A is 0.9 and the frequency of a is 0.1, the frequencies of AA, Aa and aa individuals are: 0.81, 0.18 and 0.01. This distribution is called the Hardy-Weinberg equilibrium.

Non-random mating results in a deviation from the Hardy-Weinberg distribution. Humans mate assortatively according to race; we are more likely to mate with someone of own race than another. In populations that mate this way, fewer heterozygotes are found than would be predicted under random mating (Heterozygote: An organism that has two different alleles at a locus). A decrease in heterozygotes can be the result of mate choice, or simply the result of population subdivision. Most organisms have a limited dispersal capability, so their mate will be chosen from the local population.

In bacteria

Most analyses have revealed large differences in gene content between even closely related strains. For example, comparison of the laboratory strain *Escherichia coli* K12 to both uropathogenic and enterohemorrhagic strains revealed that startlingly few genes (<40% of the total number of genes present; Fig. 12.1) were shared by these three strains (Welch et al., 2002). One interpretation is that different strains exploit somewhat different ecologies by virtue of metabolic differences imparted by different gene inventories. The collection of genes shared among members of the same species— that is, the clade-specific metagenome—has been termed the 'pan-genome'. Similar levels of variation are observed among nine genomes of *E. coli* and *Shigella* (which are essentially strains of *E. coli*). (Konstantinidis and Tiedje, 2005).

Although some genes may be more recalcitrant to transfer, genes within core genomes might have been transferred or even replaced. Such transfers can replace even highly conserved genes; e.g. lateral transfer of 16S rRNA genes has been described in both bacteria (Yap et al. 1999 and Eardly et al. 2005) and Archaea (Boucher et al. 2004).

For example, Charlebois and Doolittle (Charlebois and Doolittle, 2004) estimated that bacteria share between 100 and 150 genes, whereas only 30–50 genes appear to be shared amongst all free-living prokaryotes—much fewer than required for survival of a free-living cell. This suggests that non-orthologous replacement might be common place. More importantly, they established that, as predicted, the core genome becomes smaller, when taxa of increasing diversity are examined. The bacterial core of 125 genes is much smaller than the proteobacterial core of 1500 genes or the *E. coli* core of 3000 genes. Similarly, the genomes of pathogens *Bordatella pertussis* and *Bordatella parapertussis* differ from that of the less virulent *Bordatella bronchiseptica*, primarily owing to gene loss (Parkhill et al., 2003); this is reflected in few genes being unique to either the *B. pertussis* or *B. parapertussis* genome, and many genes lost from the *B. pertussis* genome (Fig. 12.1). Therefore, the pan-genome of some lineages might be closely approximated by the sequences of one or a few genomes. For example, near complete genomes of *Leptospirillum* and *Ferroplasma* were deduced from environmental samples found in an acid hot-spring (Tyson et al., 2004), which suggests that the pan-genomes of these specialized ecologically-restricted organisms are smaller than those of bacteria that adopt a more generalist lifestyle. For example, modification of toxin gene expression by increased promoter efficiency in *B. pertussis* contributes to the pathogenicity of this strain (Parkhill et al., 2003); such modifications accompany massive gene loss rather than gene gain (Fig. 12.1).

Comparisons of genome content in three sets of bacteria. Here, the 'pan-genome' is encompassed within the Venn diagram, and the 'core genome' is represented by the shaded region that denotes the genes shared among all three genomes. Numbers inside the Venn diagrams indicate the number of genes (and percentage of total) found to be shared among the indicated genomes; for *Buchnera*, the numbers reflect analyses without/with pseudogenes. Numbers outside the diagram indicate the number of genes in each genome and the percentage identity of the genes that encode the 23S

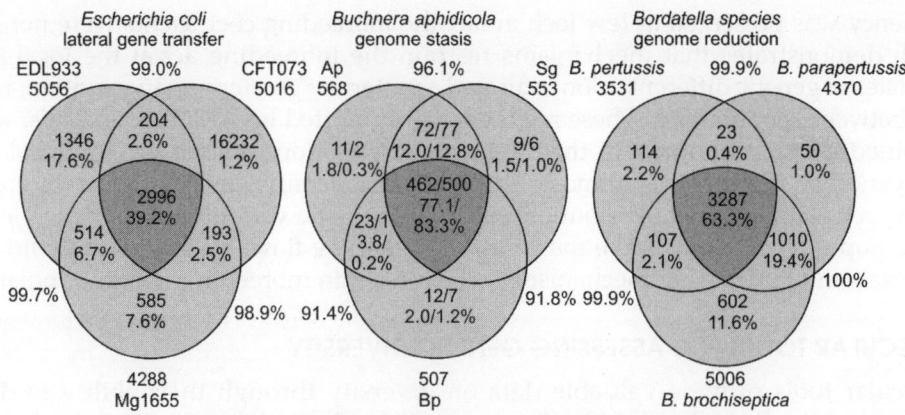

Fig. 12.1: Genome contents in three sets of bacteria

rRNA. Data are presented as reported for genomes of *Escherichia coli* (Welch., 2002), *Buchnera* and *Bordatella* lateral gene transfer, large affect of gene acquisition on gene content; genome stasis, little change in gene content; genome reduction, large affect of gene loss on gene content.

Genes that are considered to belong to the core, when closely related genomes are compared will be classified as flexible, when genomes of more distantly related organisms are compared. Several factors control the non-random patterns of gene exchange among genomes. Beyond their unequal propensities for transfer (Nakamura et al. 2004), genes are not mobilized at random. In many cases, large regions of DNA are integrated — these are denoted as genomic islands, a general term that encompasses pathogenicity, symbiosis, ecological and saprophytic islands (Hacker and Carniel., 2001). Genomic islands are typically large (tens of kilobases), are often associated with tRNAs and a linked integrase gene, and show an unusual nucleotide composition — all of which are signs of foreign origin. Genomic islands lose genes by deletion and pseudogene formation (Middendorf et al. 2004). In addition, islands contain DNA that does not contribute to purported adaptive phenotypes; e.g. a 100 kb insertion in Salmonella dedicates only 5 kb to sucrose degradation (Hochhut et al., 1997), the proposed selection for maintenance of this island (Dobrindt et al., 2004). Similarly, genes in the SPI-3 cluster can be eliminated without having any effect on pathogenicity (Blanc-Potard et al., 1999). Therefore, additional unidentified beneficial functions must be encoded in these islands to prevent the eventual loss of these genes.

Several processes affect genome evolution. First, the flow of genes between genomes is influenced both by the variability in efficacy of transfer among different classes of genes, and by the frequent transfer of large blocks of genes as genomic islands. This process results in closely related strains harboring a 'core' genome augmented by a sampling of genes from its pan-genome.

In Fungi

Urbaneilli et al., (2003) studied using allozymes and PCR fingerprinting was conducted to estimate the genetic diversity of Italian populations of two economically important cultivated fungal taxa, *Pleurotus eryngii* and *P. ferulae*. They observed that heterozygote deficiency was presented at few loci; in fact the inbreeding coefficients were not high, which demonstrates that mechanisms restrain the inbreeding act at the local level. Estimates of genetic differentiation indicated a pattern of greater variation within, rather than between, populations. These results were supported by AMOVA analysis, which attributed a low proportion of the total genetic variation to large geographical scale divergence, and indicated that most of the genetic diversity was because of differences within populations. This distribution pattern of genetic variation of *P. eryngii* and *P. ferulae* populations seems to be the result of high gene flow, by efficient basidiospore dispersal, and outcrossing mechanisms, which restrain inbreeding within populations.

MOLECULAR TOOLS FOR ASSESSING GENETIC DIVERSITY

Molecular tools provide valuable data on diversity through their ability to detect variation at the DNA level. Identification is of fundamental importance in diversity studies in a variety of different ways. A number of different techniques are available for identifying genetic differences between organisms. Protein polymorphisms were the first markers used for genetic studies in livestock. However, the number of polymorphic loci that can be assayed, and the level of polymorphisms observed at the loci are often low, which greatly limits their application in genetic diversity studies. Recently, various molecular techniques have contributed to our understanding of genetic diversity, evolution and pathogenesis, e.g. RFLP, AFLP, FAME and RAPD, etc.

Restriction Fragment Length Polymorphism (RFLP)

All organisms have numerous differences in their genomic DNA sequence and therefore, are genotypically distinct. This difference results in a restriction fragment length polymorphism. This can be detected by southern hybridization after running agarose gel electrophoresis. Hybridization analysis is carried out using probe that spans the region of interest. The probe hybridizes to the relevant region, 'lighting up' the appropriate restriction fragments on the resulting autoradiograph. If an RFLP is present then it will be clearly visible on the autoradiograph (Southern, 1979). Thus RFLP is used as a major tool to identify the genetic diversity within and between species (Old and Primrosed, 1998) (Fig. 12.2).

Random Amplified Polymorphic DNA (RAPD)

The invention of PCR (polymerase chain reaction) is a milestone in the development of molecular techniques. PCR results in the selective amplification of a chosen region of a DNA molecule. Random amplification of DNA with short primer by PCR is a useful technique in phylogenetics. The important point is the banding pattern seen, when the products of PCR with random primers are electrophoresed in a reflection of the overall structure of the DNA molecule used as the template. If the starting material is total cell DNA then the banding pattern represents the organization of the cell's genome. Differences between the genomes of two organisms can be measured with RAPD. Two closely related organisms would be expected to yield more similar banding patterns than two organisms that are distant in evolutionary terms (Miesfeld, 1999). Moreover, this technique requires only small piece of animal tissue or blood, as the extracted DNA can be amplified million times using PCR (Fig. 12.3).

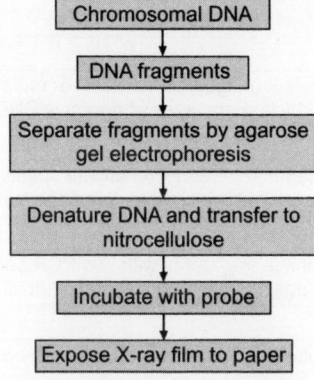

Fig. 12.2: Protocol of RFLP

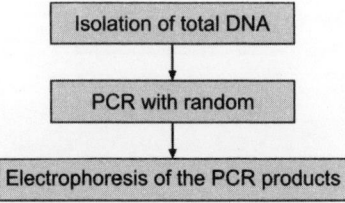

Fig. 12.3: Protocol of RAPD

Amplified Polymorphic Length Polymorphism (AFLP)

AFLP analysis is able to detect high levels of polymorphism and has high repeatability and speed of analysis. These markers have a very high diversity index, resulting in a limited number of primer combinations required to screen a whole genome and has been applied to develop a system for the fingerprinting of an organism (Faccioli et al. 1999) and for map expansion (Castiglioni et al. 1998). Vos et al. (1995) described the AFLP technique as being based on the detection of restriction fragments by PCR amplification and argued that the reliability of the RFLP technique is combined with the power of the PCR technique. AFLPs provide high levels of resolution to allow delineation of complex genetic structures. AFLPs are fragments of DNA that have been amplified using directed primers from restriction digested genomic DNA (Matthes et al., 1998; Karp et al., 1997) (Fig. 12.4).

FAME (Fatty Acid Methyl Ester) Analysis

Another approach for assessing diversity involves analysis of FAME profiles. This technique has been nick-named FAME or fatty acid methyl ester. For actual analysis, fatty acids extracted from bulk lipid of a bacterial culture grown under standardized condition, are chemically modified to form their corresponding methyl esters; these volatile derivatives are identified by gas chromatography. A computerized llist of types and amount of fatty acids from the unknown bacterium is then compared with a database containing the fatty acid profiles of thousands of reference bacteria grown under the same condition, and the best matches to that of the unknown selected (Fig. 12.5).

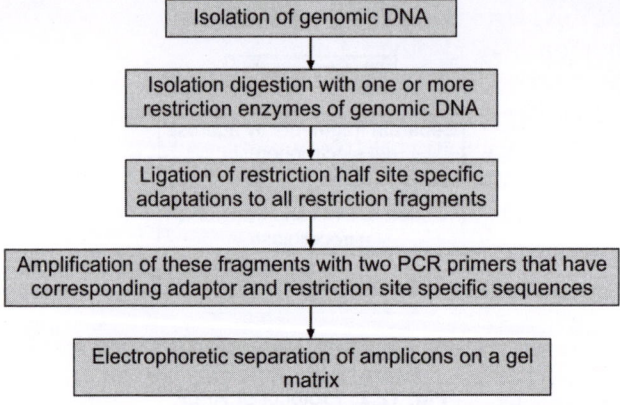

Fig. 12.4: Protocol of AFLP

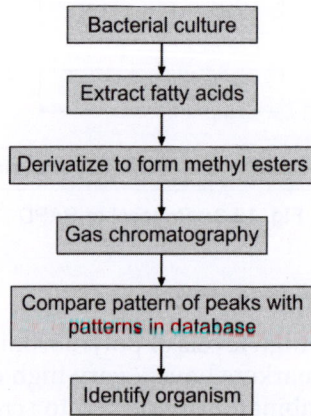

Fig. 12.5: Protocol of FAME

Microsatellites

Microsatellites, alternatively known as simple sequence repeats (SSRs), short tandem repeats (STRs) or simple sequence length polymorphisms (SSLPs), are tandem repeats of sequence units generally less than 5 bp in length (Bruford and Wayne, 1993). These markers appear to be hypervariable, in addition to which their codominance and reproducibility make them ideal for genome mapping, as well as for population genetic studies (Dayanandan et al., 1998). One common example of a microsatellite is a (CA) repeat (Fig. 12.6), where *n* is variable between alleles. These markers often present high levels of inter-and intraspecific polymorphism, particularly when tandem repeats number ten or greater. CA nucleotide repeats are very frequent in human and other genomes, and present every few thousand base pairs. InterSSRs are a variant of the RAPD technique, although the higher annealing temperatures probably mean that they are more rigorous than RAPDs. Chloroplast microsatellites (cpSSRs) are similar to nuclear microsatellites but the repeat is usually only 1 bp, i.e. (T) *n* (Provan et al., 1999). Microsatellites owe their variability to an increased rate of mutation compared to other neutral regions of DNA. These high rates of mutation can be explained most frequently by slipped strand mispairing (slippage) during DNA replication on a single DNA double helix. Mutation may also occur during recombination during meiosis. Some errors in slippage are rectified by proofreading mechanisms within the nucleus, but some mutations can escape repair. The size of the repeat unit, the number of repeats, the presence of variant repeats and the frequency of transcription in the area of the DNA repeat are the factors responsible for generating polymorphism. Larger changes in repeat number are though to be the result of processes such as unequal crossing over (Strand et al., 1993).

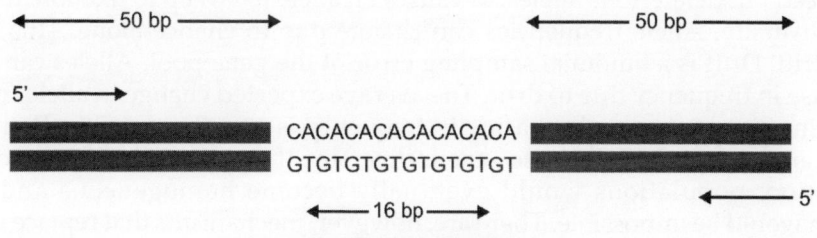

Fig. 12.6: Microsatellite

Such differences are detected on polyacrylamide gels (Fig. 12.7.), where repeat lengths migrate different distances according to their sizes.

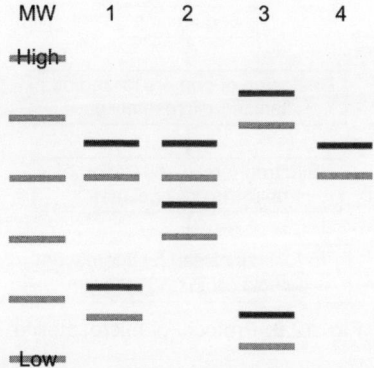

Fig. 12.7: Polymorphism in microsatellite

Protocol

The microsatellite protocol is simple, once primers for SSRs have been designed. The first stage is a PCR, depending upon the method of detection, one of the primers is fluorescently or radioactively labelled. The PCR products are separated on high resolution polyacrylamide gels, and the products detected with a fluorescence detector (e.g. automated sequencer) or an X-ray film. The investigator can determine the size of the PCR product and thus how many times the short nucleotide was repeated for each allele.

MECHANISM THAT INCREASE AND DECREASE THE GENETIC DIVERSITY

The cellular machinery that copies DNA sometimes makes mistakes. These mistakes alter the sequence of a gene. This is called a mutation. Most mutations that have any phenotypic effect are deleterious. Only a very small percentage of mutations are beneficial. A change in environment can cause previously neutral alleles to have selective values; in the short-term evolution can run on "stored" variation and thus is independent of mutation rate. Other mechanisms can also contribute selectable variation. Recombination creates new combinations of alleles (or new alleles) by joining sequences with separate microevolutionary histories within a population. Gene flow can also supply the gene pool with variants but the ultimate source of these variants is mutation. Natural selection can maintain or deplete genetic variation. When selection acts to weed out deleterious alleles, or causes an allele to sweep to fixation, it depletes genetic diversity. Allele frequencies can change due to chance alone. This is called genetic drift. Drift is a binomial sampling error of the gene pool. Alleles can increase or decrease in frequency due to drift. The average expected change in allele frequency is zero, since increasing or decreasing in frequency is equally probable. Both natural selection and genetic drift decrease genetic diversity. If they were the only mechanisms of evolution, populations would eventually become homogeneous and further evolution would be impossible. There are, however, mechanisms that replace variation depleted by selection and drift, e.g. mutation.

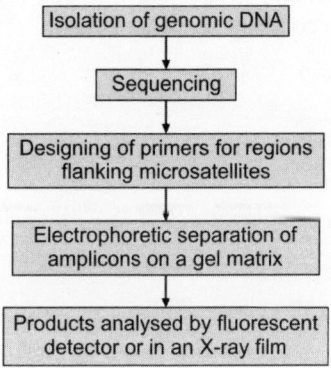

Fig. 12.8: Protocol of microsatellite

CONCLUSION

All living organisms carry a genetic blueprint. This is so regardless of whether they are plants, animals, or microorganisms, whether they are short- or long-lived, and whether they reproduce sexually or clonally. Therefore, to the extent that restoration deals with living organisms, genetics are part of the picture. Organisms exist in environments that vary in time and over space. Such variation is often described in terms of the natural or historic range of variability (NRV, HRV) in environmental conditions such as weather, disturbance events, resource availability, population sizes of competitors, etc. (White and Walker, 1997). If a group of organisms (say, a population of species X) were to live in a completely stable physical and biological environment, then a relatively narrow range of phenotypes might be optimally adapted to those conditions. Under these circumstances, species X would benefit more by maintaining a narrow range of genotypes adapted to prevailing conditions, and allele frequencies might eventually attain equilibrium. By contrast, if the environment is patchy, unpredictable over time, or includes a wide and changing variety of diseases, predators, and parasites, then subtle differences among individuals increase the probability that some individuals and not others will survive to reproduce, i.e. the traits are "exposed to selection." Since differences among individuals are determined at least partly by genotype, population genetic theory predicts (and empirical observation confirms) that in variable environments a broader range of genetic variation (higher heterozygosity) will persist (Cohen 1966, Chesson 1985, Tuljapurkar 1989, Tilman 1999).

Examples of traits with a genetic basis for tolerance of environmental variation important in restoration work include tolerance of freezing, drought or inundation, high or low light availability, salinity, heavy metals, soil nutrient deficiencies, and extreme soil pH values in plants; resilience to fluctuating temperature, dissolved oxygen, and nutrient availability in aquatic organisms; and resistance to novel diseases in all groups of organisms (Huenneke, 1991). For example, if all individuals in a population are the same genotype with limited drought tolerance, then a single climatic event may destroy the entire population. Plant populations often include individuals with a range of flowering or emergence times. A diverse array of genotypes appears to be especially important in disease resistance (Schoen and Brown, 1993; McArdle, 1996). Genetically uniform populations (such as highly inbred crops) are famously vulnerable to diseases and pathogens, which can (and do) decimate populations in which all individuals are equally vulnerable. Such uniformity also predisposes a population to transmit disease from one individual to another — instead of having isolated diseased individuals, nearly every individual may be exposed to disease by direct contact or proximity. More diverse populations are more likely to include individuals resistant to specific diseases; moreover, infected individuals occur at lower density, and thus diseases or pathogens may move more slowly through the population. Genetic variation is a factor in competition among individuals in real ecological communities. Finally, genetic variation holds the key to the ability of populations and species to persist over evolutionary time through changing environments (Freeman and Herron, 1998).

REFERENCES

1. Blanc-Potard AB, Solomon F, Kayser J, et al. 1999. The SPI-3 pathogenicity island of Salmonella enterica. *J Bacteriol* 181: 998–1004.

2. Boucher Y, Douady CJ, Sharma AK, et al. 2004. Intragenomic heterogeneity and intergenomic recombination among haloarchaeal rRNA genes. *J Bacteriol*, 186: 3980–3990.

3. Bruford MW, Wayne RK. 1993. Microsatellites and their application to population genetic studies. *Current Opinion in Genetics and Development*, 3: 939–943.

4. Castiglioni P, Pozzi C, Heun, M, et al. 1998. An AFLP-based procedure for the efficient mapping of mutations and DNA probes in barley. *Genetics*, 149: 2039–2056.

5. Charlebois RL, Doolittle WF. 2004. Computing prokaryotic gene ubiquity: rescuing the core from extinction. *Genome Res*, 14: 2469–2477.

6. Chesson Peter L. 1985. Coexistence of competitors in spatially and temporally varying environments: A look at the combined effects of different sorts of variability. *Theoretical Population Biology* 28: 263–287.

7. Cohen, D. (1966). Optimising reproduction in a randomly varying environment. *Journal of Theoretical Biology* 12: 119–129.

8. Dayanandan S, Rajora, O.P. and Bawa, K.S. (1998). Isolation and characterisation of microsatellites in trembling aspen (Populus tremuloides). *Theoretical and Applied Genetics*, 96: 950–956.

9. Dobrindt U, Hochhut B, Hentschel U, Hacker J. (2004). Genomic islands in pathogenic and environmental microorganisms. *Nat Rev Microbiol*, 2: 414–424.

10. Eardly BD, Nour SM, van Berkum P, Selander RK. (2005). Rhizobial 16S rRNA and dnaK genes: mosaicism and the uncertain phylogenetic placement of Rhizobium galegae. *Appl Environ Microbiol* 71: 1328–1335.

11. Faccioli P., Pecchioni, N., Stanca, A.M. and Terzi, V. (1999). Amplified fragment length polymorphism (AFLP) markers for barley malt fingerprinting. *J. Cereal Sci.*, 29: 257–260.

12. Freeman, Scott, and Jon C. Herron. (1998). Evolutionary analysis. *Upper Saddle River*, New Jersey: Prentice-Hall.

13. Groom, M.J., Meffe, G.K. and Carroll, C.R. (2006) *Principles of Conservation Biology* (3rd ed.). Sunderland, MA: Sinauer Associates.

14. Hacker J, Carniel E. (2001).Ecological fitness, genomic islands and bacterial pathogenicity. A Darwinian view of the evolution of microbes. *EMBO Rep*, 2: 376–381.

15. Hochhut B, Jahreis K, Lengeler JW, Schmid K. (1997). CTnscr 94, a conjugative transposon found in enterobacteria. *J Bacteriol* 179: 2097–2102.

16. Huenneke, Laura F. (1991). Ecological implications of genetic variation in plant populations. In *Genetics and Conservation of Rare Plants*, edited by D. A. Falk and K. E. Holsinger. New York: Oxford University Press.

17. Karp, A., Kresovich, S., Bhat, K.V., Ayand, W.G. and Hodgkin, T. (1997). Molecular tools in plant genetic resources conservation: A guide to the technologies. IPGRI Technical Bulletin No. 2, International Plant Genetic Resources Institute, Rome, Italy. Available at http://198.93.227.125/publicat/techbull/TB2.pdf.

18. Konstantinidis KT, Tiedje JM. (2005). Genomic insights that advance the species definition for prokaryotes. *Proc Natl Acad Sci USA*, 102:2567–2572.

19. Lankau, Richard, (2007). Study: Loss Of Genetic Diversity Threatens Species Diversity

20. Matthes, M.C., Daly, A. and Edwards, K.J. (1998). Amplified fragment length polymorphism (AFLP). In: Karp A, Isaac PG, Ingram DS (eds.). *Molecular Tools for Screening Biodiversity*. Chapman and Hall, London, pp. 183–190.

21. McArdle, B. H. (1996). Levels of evidence in studies of competition, predation, and disease. *New Zealand Journal of Ecology* 20: 7–15.

22. Middendorf B, Hochhut B, Leipold K, Dobrindt U, Blum-Oehler G, Hacker J. (2004). Instability of pathogenicity islands in uropathogenic Escherichia coli 536. *J Bacteriol*, 186: 3086–3096.

23. Miesfeld R.L. (1999). Rapid amplification of DNA. In *Applied Molecular Genetics*. A John Wiley and Sons, INC., Publication.

24. Nakamura Y, Itoh T, Matsuda H, Gojobori T. (2004). Biased biological functions of horizontally transferred genes in prokaryotic genomes. *Nat Genet*, 36: 760–766.

25. Old, R.W. and Primrose, S.B. (1998). Principles of gene manipulation. *An Introduction to Genetic Engineering*. Fifth Edition. Blackwell Science Limite.

26. Parkhill J, Sebaihia M, Preston A, Murphy LD, Thomson N, Harris DE, Holden MT, Churcher CM, Bentley SD, Mungall KL et al . (2003).: Comparative analysis of the genome sequences of Bordetella pertussis, Bordetella parapertussis and Bordetella bronchiseptica. *Nat Genet*, 35: 32–40.

27. Proven, J., Russell, J.R., Booth, A. and Powell, W. (1999). Polymorphic chloroplast simple sequence repeat primers for systematic and population studies in the genus Hordeum. *Molecular Ecology*, 8: 505–511.

28. Schoen, D. J., and A. H. D. Brown. (1993). Conservation of allelic richness in wild crop relatives is aided by assessment of genetic markers. *Proc. National Academy of Science* (US) 90: 10623–10627.

29. Southern, E.M. (1979). Gel electrophoresis of restriction fragments. *Methods Enzymol.*, 68: 152–76.d.

30. Strand, M., Prolla, T.A., Liskay, R.M. and Petes, T.D. (1993). Destabilisation of tracts of simple repetitive DNA in yeast by mutations affecting DNA mismatch repair. *Nature*, 365: 274–276.

31. Tilman, David. (1999). The ecological consequences of changes in biodiversity: A search for general principles. *Ecology* 80: 1455–1474.

32. Tisdell, C. (2003). "Socioeconomic causes of loss of animal genetic diversity: Analysis and assessment". *Ecological Economics* 45 (3): 365–376.

33. Tuljapurkar, Shripad. (1989). An uncertain life: Demography in random environments. *Theoretical Population Biology* 35: 227–294.

34. Tyson GW, Chapman J, Hugenholtz P, Allen EE, Ram RJ, Richardson PM, Solovyev VV, Rubin EM, Rokhsar DS, Banfield JF. (2004). Community structure and metabolism through reconstruction of microbial genomes from the environment. *Nature*, 428: 37–43.

35. Urbanelli S, Rosa V Della, Fanelli C, Fabbri A A and Reverberi M (2003). Genetic diversity and population structure of the Italian fungi belonging to the taxa *Pleurotus eryngii* (DC.:Fr.) Quèl and *P. ferulae* (DC.: Fr.) Quèl. *Heredity* 90, 253–259.

36. Vos, P., Hogers, R., Bleeker, M., Reijans, M., van de Lee, T., Hornes, M., Frijters, A., Pot, J., Peleman, J., Kuiper, M. and Zabeau, M. (1995). AFLP: a new technique for DNA fingerprinting. *Nucleic Acids Research*, 23: 4407–4414.

37. Welch RA, Burland V, Plunkett G III, Redford P, Roesch P, Rasko D, Buckles EL, Liou SR, Boutin A, Hackett J et al. (2002). Extensive mosaic structure revealed by the complete genome White, Peter S., and Joan L. Walker. (1997). Approximating nature's variation: selecting and using reference information in restoration ecology. *Restoration Ecology* 5 (4): 338–349.

38. Yap WH, Zhang Z, Wang Y.(1999).Distinct types of rRNA operons exist in the genome of the Actinomycete Thermomonospora chromogena and evidence for horizontal transfer of an entire rRNA operon. *J Bacteriol*, 181: 5201–5209.

Index

Reader's Note

Reader's Note